Principles of economic appraisal in health care

M. F. Drummond
Lecturer in Economics
Health Services Management Centre
University of Birmingham

Oxford New York Toronto Melbourne

OXFORD UNIVERSITY PRESS

1980

Oxford University Press, Walton Street, Oxford OX2 6DP
London Glasgow New York Toronto
Delhi Bombay Calcutta Madras Karachi
Kuala Lumpur Singapore Hong Kong Tokyo
Nairobi Dar Es Salaam Cape Town
Melbourne Wellington
and associate companies in
Beirut Berlin Ibadan Mexico City

Published in the United States
by Oxford University Press, New York

British Library Cataloguing in Publication Data
   Drummond, M F
   Principles of economic appraisal in
   health care.—Oxford medical publications).
   1. Medical care—Great Britain
   —Cost effectiveness
   I. Title   II. Series
   338.4'3   RA410.55.G7   80-40343

ISBN 0-19-261273-5

Filmset in 'Monophoto' by Eta Services (Typesetters) Ltd., Beccles, Suffolk
Printed in Great Britain by Lowe & Brydone Printers Limited,
Thetford, Norfolk

To Margaret

Foreword

Alan Williams, Professor of Economics, University of York

One cannot but sympathize with clinicians and other health service professionals who feel that with so many pressures upon them they might at least be spared the distasteful task of having to think about efficiency, and the husbanding of scarce resources, on top of all their other problems. It is, therefore, not surprising that some of them sit tight, hoping that the pressure to 'economize' will go away if simply outfaced, or, better still, that someone else will sort it all out, to their complete satisfaction, if simply instructed to do so. A little calm reflection soon dispels both illusions, however, and with the growing realization that economic and financial stringency is likely both to intensify and persist, many have reluctantly concluded that if health services are to respond rationally and effectively then clinicians, medical researchers, and other health service professionals, need to understand, and collaborate with, economists (and vice-versa, of course) in reaching a deeper understanding of the problem of setting, and implementing, priorities.

Economics is about choice, and choice involves evaluation (or appraisal), and this project was stimulated by a desire to bridge the gap between the notion of evaluation which underlies much clinical research, and the notion of evaluation which underlies health economics research. The initiative came from the Medical Research Council and the Social Science Research Council in the U.K., whose initial interest was in testing how far techniques such as cost–benefit analysis could be used to establish priorities within their respective research programmes in the health field. It soon became obvious, however, that until more was known about the costs and benefits of many existing clinical practices, and proposed changes therein, it would be extremely difficult to tackle the higher level task of choosing between them.

Among the major obstacles to the initiation of such evaluative work (even amongst those who were already convinced of its *potential* value) was (a) a lack of appreciation of what was involved in formulating problems in a manner appropriate for economic appraisal, (b) an unwillingness to make the apparently superhuman effort required to master the rather forbidding jargon of the typical economic treatise on this subject, (c) a fear that if some fanatical and incomprehensible economists were turned loose on some piece of clinical evaluation, the whole project would get totally out of control, and (d) nagging doubts about what (if anything) was likely to be achieved at the end of the day that could not be achieved by the tried and tested methods of one's own discipline (perhaps with a little help from a 'tame' accountant!).

Rather than embark on yet another exercise in salesmanship, asserting again our belief in the importance and relevance of cost–benefit and cost effectiveness techniques to both clinical and health services research, we thought it might be better to adopt a different approach, namely, that of explaining, step-by-step, what would be involved, so that those who are (understandably) sceptical about such claims could judge for themselves whether there really is anything in all this for them. This volume is therefore, an Intelligent Child's Guide to Economic Appraisal in Health Care (though admittedly for a rather mature, and perhaps even somewhat precocious, child!).

Since telling people what ought to be done is frequently less convincing than showing them what has actually been done so far, we decided to offer the reader, in addition, a sizeable selection of studies which collectively cover a wide range of applications of economic appraisal to health care alternatives. (These are given in the companion volume, *Studies in economic appraisal in health care.*) One objective in so doing is to stimulate the reader's imagination. It also demonstrates that there is a great deal of useful and commendable work which falls far short of perfection, for 'ideal' evaluation is no more readily attainable in the economic field than it is elsewhere. Evaluation is hard work and is bound to be constrained in practice by data problems, uncooperative respondents, lack of time and money, and sometimes by the failure of the researcher to see at the beginning of a project that some variable is crucial which, with hindsight, proves to be a serious omission from the study. Economic appraisal is just as vulnerable in these respects as is any other kind of evaluation.

One could, therefore, say that this guide has been offered as an attempt to 'demythologize' micro-economic analysis, not only because we think the basic ideas should be communicable to intelligent beings in other disciplines, but also as an act of reciprocity for the efforts that many health service professionals have put in over the years in trying patiently to explain in simple terms some of the otherwise impenetrable mysteries of medicine. Interdisciplinary communication in this field may be difficult, but it is also essential if there is to be a fruitful cooperation between economists and others on tackling the problems faced by health services all over the world.

Preface

This guide is produced for non-economists with an interest in economic appraisal in the field of health care. It is primarily for those who already recognize a need for such appraisal, and therefore the emphasis has been on pointing out the essential features of economic analysis, rather than trying to convert others to this particular way of thinking. However, I have devoted a little space to the latter activity in Chapter 1. Conversely, it is possible that after reading this guide, a few of the converted will be left in despair. If this is the case, then I have failed.

In particular, I had two groups in mind when producing the guide. The first of these consists of those medical researchers, epidemiologists, clinicians, and other health professionals already engaged in multidisciplinary research, or wishing to add an economic perspective to their appraisals of health service alternatives. As the book has evolved, I have become increasingly aware of the difficulties *and dangers* of writing 'cookbooks'. Therefore I would hope that one of the outcomes of reading the guide is that the non-economist is *more* (rather than less) likely to seek professional economic advice. At a number of points in the book I have skated over issues which themselves have generated large quantities of literature. I have opted for this course mainly in the interests of brevity, but partly because some of the issues remain unresolved. Nevertheless I hope that for this group the guide will at least:

1. Enable the non-economist to appreciate more fully the essential features of economic appraisal, so that (technical) research design and data collection may be tailored accordingly;
2. Facilitate the early stages of the dialogue between the non-economist and his economist colleague or adviser (although I recognize that the discussions concerning a particular appraisal will soon go beyond the point where a general text can be of help).

Second, I set out to help those whose planning or managerial responsibilities require them to undertake a critical assessment of existing economic appraisals. For this group, I hope that the guide:

1. Enables them to pinpoint particular shortcomings in existing work in the particular area under study.
2. Enables them to appreciate what would be required to improve upon existing work in order that (say) the planning question in hand could be answered.

In short, I would hope that the guide contributes both to the understanding (by non-economists) of the methods of appraisal economists have used to date and to improvements in economic appraisals carried out in the future.

M.F.D.

Birmingham
June 1980

Acknowledgements

This book and its companion volume, *Studies in economic appraisal in health care*, were produced as a result of a review of the cost effectiveness and cost–benefit literature in health care which was commissioned and financed by the Social Science Research Council (SSRC). This was undertaken during my employment as a Research Fellow at the Institute of Social and Economic Research (ISER), University of York, and formed part of the Institute's research programme in health economics.

My major debt is to Alan Williams and to Ken Wright of ISER, the supervisors of the project, who offered help and encouragement throughout. My other main debt is to all those economists and non-economists who read and commented on earlier drafts. Needless to say, none of these is responsible for any remaining errors.

Although they were not directly concerned with this project, I would like also to record my thanks to Tony Culyer, Bob Lavers, Alan Maynard, Arthur Walker, and Jack Wiseman for their help and advice during my stay at York. Finally, I would like to thank Miss Barbara Dodds and the Secretarial Staff at ISER for their efficient work.

Contents

1
Introduction

1.1. Appraisal in health care

The day-to-day operation of any health service requires numerous choices between alternative courses of action. Choices may be made in two broad contexts; first, when it has to be decided what particular course of action is best for a particular patient or client, and second, when it has to be decided what course of action is best in the planning of health services for a whole community or various groups of people. It is with the latter set of choices that this book is mainly concerned. That is not to say that the guide is of no interest to clinical practitioners, since many of them are involved in evaluation of current practice with a view to future improvement of services, or more directly in the planning of services, through their attendance on medical committees and planning teams. In addition, some practitioners will find that many of the ideas expressed below are pertinent to their present clinical actions. After all, in giving treatment or advice, most practitioners will feel a responsibility not only for the health of the individual being treated at that moment, but also for the health of those waiting for treatment. Therefore, it could be said that the distinction made above is somewhat false, since all of those involved in the making of health care choices are really having to make them for a group of individuals. The only factor that varies is the size of the group, the largest group to be considered being the whole community.†

Some choices for the community may be between objectives (e.g.

---

† The application of economic concepts in the clinical context is discussed in Appendix 1. It should be noted that, given limited resources, doing one's best for the group of patients/clients under one's control may not be the same as giving each client (taken individually) as much care as one would like. For this reason, the extent to which individual practitioners allow resource constraints to influence their behaviour remains a matter for individual clinical judgement and in that context the role of economic analysis is to make clear the implications of different ways of responding to that dilemma.

is it better to reduce waiting time for orthopaedic surgery or to expand community care for the mentally handicapped?). Other choices may be between different means of achieving a given objective (e.g. what is the best mix of institutional and community care for the elderly? Is it better to treat some minor conditions by day-case surgery or by traditional in-patient management?). In fact the delivery of any form of health care requires answers to be given to the following questions: whom to treat; when to begin treatment; how to treat; where to treat; how much treatment to offer?†

Appraisal is concerned with the analysis of alternative courses of action with a view to assisting choice. While there is no simple, single basis for making community-wide choices, it is possible to identify a number of relevant criteria for choice. One such criterion is *economic efficiency*.

1.2. The criterion of economic efficiency

The community engages in health care activities in order to derive benefits for its members. The same is true for other activities, such as the provision of education and housing. The need for efficiency in all these activities arises from the fact that there will never be enough resources to satisfy human wants completely. (Economists refer to this as the notion of *scarcity*.) Given scarcity, it follows that use of resources in a given beneficial activity inevitably involves a sacrifice. That is, the community forgoes the opportunity to use the same resources in other beneficial activities.

The economist's concept of *cost* stems from this notion of alternative uses for scarce resources. The cost of a unit of a resource is the benefit that would be derived from using it in its best alternative use.‡ This concept should be contrasted with a strictly financial concept of cost, which relates to the cash outlays for units of the resource. It will be seen later (Chapter 4) that in some instances the economic, and the financial estimates of the cost of health treatments may coincide, but this will frequently not be the case. So, it is important to bear in mind throughout the book this fundamental conceptual distinction.

---

† Throughout the book, the word 'treatment' will be used in the widest possible sense. It will be taken to include all forms of patient (or client) management, not just that administered by doctors. In addition, preventive and 'caring' regimens will be classed as 'treatments'.

‡ Hence the economist's term, 'opportunity cost'.

Adoption of the criterion of *economic efficiency* implies that choices in health care should be made so as to derive the maximum total benefit from the resources at the community's disposal. In practice, this involves the appraisal of health care alternatives through the calculation of the amount by which the benefits generated exceed the costs (sacrifices) incurred. Therefore, it is implicit in the efficiency criterion that a given treatment or procedure cannot be preferred over another solely on the basis of being more beneficial, or solely on the basis of being less costly. The choice will depend on both relative benefits *and* relative costs. After all, the costs merely represent benefits forgone elsewhere.

While the basic notion of maximizing the total benefit to the community for the use of its resources is unlikely to have many dissenters, it can be seen that the discussion of efficiency raises many issues. Who are, or what constitutes, the community? What are the benefits arising from health care programmes? How are the benefits and costs estimated, and by whom? Is it important to know the *distribution* of the benefits of health care programmes amongst different groups within the community?

Most of these issues will be dealt with later. However, it is worth clearing up two popular misconceptions at this stage. First, the benefit to the community of a particular activity is merely the sum of the benefits accruing to individuals in the community.† That is, the community does not constitute a 'person' in its own right. Second, the economist's concept of benefits is very wide. It includes not only the benefits derived from patients (or clients) being able to return to work (and hence add to the nation's production) but also the benefits derived from being healthy *per se*. It is probably best to view the former as merely one component of the latter. Economists are doubtless mainly to blame for the widespread misconception that the only benefits they are interested in are those which relate to people's productive capabilities. It will be seen in the review of existing work that economic analysis has indeed concentrated on valuing these benefits. This is not to say that economists regard healthiness *per se* as being unimportant, rather it reflects the difficulties they experience in measuring and valuing this category of benefit. This is a key issue which will arise a number of times throughout the book.

† See Appendix 2.

Despite the potential difficulties, it can be seen that efficiency provides a wider framework for choice between alternatives in health care than that provided by technical (medical) appraisal alone. At best, medical appraisal can indicate some of the desirable and undesirable effects of a treatment, but until it is complemented by an analysis of resource costs it can tell us nothing about the benefits forgone.

1.3. Is economic appraisal all that is required?

At this point one might be tempted to ask whether economic appraisal, properly carried out, provides the answers to all questions of choice in health care. The answer is 'no', and for two reasons. First, economic appraisal is highly dependent upon the underlying technical appraisal. For instance, the assessment of the costs and benefits of alternative health treatments requires details of the range of feasible alternatives, the resource requirements of each alternative and the results (or outcomes) produced by each alternative. Here the economist is very much in the hands of the relevant technical experts. Economic appraisal should, therefore, be viewed as a complement to medical (and other technical) appraisal, rather than as a substitute for it. For this reason, economists have just as much interest as others in making sure that the *effectiveness* of treatments is properly assessed. (For a discussion of the assessment of effectiveness see Cochrane (1972).)† The review will show that on occasions 'good' economics has been superimposed upon 'bad' medical appraisal. (It is equally possible, of course, to find bad economics associated with good medical appraisal.)

The second reason why economic appraisal cannot provide all the answers is that efficiency may not be the only criterion for judging health care alternatives. *Equity* is often suggested as another relevant criterion. (This is, of course, related to the distribution question, alluded to in §1.2.) Equity can prove to be a very slippery concept. For instance, in health care one could have several notions

---

† Cochrane defines an effective treatment as one which alters the natural history of the disease. It is assumed here that this definition would include placebos and treatments which prevent or slow down deterioration of a given condition. One could even extend the definition to include those treatments which do not alter the natural history of the disease but provide relief and comfort to patients or their relatives. Defined in this way one can consider the assessment of effectiveness to be an important step along the road towards the assessment of efficiency.

of equity: equal access to care by geographical area; equal shares between client groups; equal access irrespective of income; and equal access for equal need. In the past, economists have given relatively little attention to equity considerations. However, there are a number of ways of handling situations where one has more than one criterion. One way would be to decide (say, on equity grounds) upon the funds to be allocated to given groups by way of the political process. For example, in the UK, proposals have been put forward to allocate funds between Regions and between client groups (DHSS 1976 a,b; SHHD 1976, 1977). Once the broad allocations have been decided upon, one could then adopt the efficiency criterion in choosing between alternative patterns of care for each group. More generally, one way round the problem of multiple criteria would be to allow (say) equity considerations to act as a constraint on how far one would pursue efficiency. That is, one would appraise alternatives in accordance with the efficiency criterion, selecting the most efficient alternative, subject to certain equity considerations being met.†

However, in view of the additional complications which equity considerations introduce into the analysis it may be prudent at the first stage to concentrate on efficiency and to view economic appraisal merely as an *aid* to decision-making, albeit an important and hitherto neglected one (see Fig. 1.1).

1.4. The plan of the book

The object of this volume is to give an outline of the basic steps involved in undertaking an economic appraisal of health care alternatives. In Chapter 2, the economist's notions of costs and benefits are explored in more detail. The aim is to give the reader an early sight of the likely requirements for an assessment of economic efficiency.

Chapters 3, 4, 5, and 6 discuss in more detail the various steps in undertaking an economic appraisal (see Fig. 1.2). Chapter 3 deals with the problems of setting up a study. It is stressed that it is important to be clear on the precise question that the study is designed to answer. It will be seen that the study question de-

---

† It is worth noting that some economists adopt a wider definition of efficiency in which distributional (or equity) objectives are included. This is often referred to as *grand efficiency*.

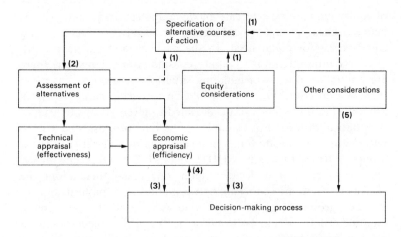

Fig. 1.1. The place of economic appraisal in the decision-making process. Key: (1) all the criteria (effectiveness, efficiency, equity, etc.) influence the original specification of alternative courses of action; (2) once the alternatives are specified they are explicitly appraised on technical and economic grounds; (3) efficiency and equity considerations are the direct inputs into the decision-making process. Technical considerations enter via efficiency only, not directly; (4) values generated by the decision-making process may be fed into the economic evaluation; (5) other factors may be taken into account when making a decision; for example, the existence of 'political' pressures, or the thought that the management structure may not be able to cope with the proposed change. These factors should not be regarded as excuses for inaction, and indeed, closer examination may show them to be part of the efficiency or equity calculus. For instance, 'political' pressures may exist because a section of the community believes that certain measures are inequitable. On the other hand, some pressures may be the result of inadequate attention being paid to consultation, either with the work-force or with the community at large. One could view the devotion of scarce resources to the necessary consultation and provision of information as part of the costs of a particular course of action, thereby influencing whether or not it would be efficient to select that alternative.

Fig. 1.2. (*opposite*) Stages in economic appraisal. Key: (1) A stimulus enters the decision-making process. This could be technical (discovery of a new technique), financial (a change in the budget or money outlays), or political (representations from a pressure group); (2) a question is formulated for study. This leads to, or is already, a statement of alternatives (Chapter 3); (3) the statement of alternatives is conditioned by the technical possibilities available; (4) technical appraisal forms the basis for the measurement of costs and benefits (Chapter 4); (5) decision-maker's values are sometimes used in the decision-making process

(*cont. opposite*)

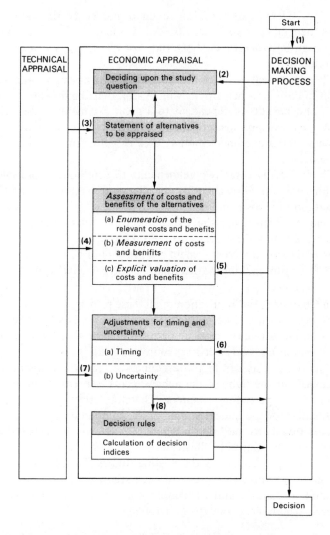

(Chapter 4); (6) decision-makers may specify the discount rate to be used in the adjustment for differential timing of costs and benefits (Chapter 5); (7) some of the uncertainty in costs and benefits arises from uncertainty in the underlying technology. Therefore, some of the estimates obtained in the technical appraisal (e.g. variation in medical outcome) have a direct bearing on the adjustments made here (Chapter 5); (8) the information arising from the economic appraisal can either go direct to the decision-makers, or can be summarized through the calculation of a decision index (Chapter 6).

termines the type of appraisal required and hence the method of assessment of costs and benefits. The two major types of economic appraisal, *cost–benefit analysis* and *cost effectiveness analysis*, are introduced.

Chapter 4 deals with the enumeration, measurement, and valuation of costs and benefits. It will be seen that the measurement of costs and benefits is dependent to a great extent upon the underlying technical appraisal of the alternative courses of action. The difficult, and sometimes emotive, area of valuation is discussed in some detail.

Chapter 5 discusses two refinements to economic appraisals in health care, the allowance for the differential timing of, and the uncertainty in, costs and benefits.

Chapter 6 discusses the use of decision rules in cost–benefit studies and how these relate to the taking of decisions. Here it is stressed further that cost–benefit studies should be seen only as an *aid* to decision-making, rather than as the total basis for arriving at a decision.

In Chapter 7, the application of all these principles is discussed in the context of four case studies. These draw on existing published work and illustrate the extra complexities required in the analysis as the question for study becomes more complex.

Finally, in Chapter 8, the usefulness of economic appraisal is discussed, in the light of the achievements and inadequacies outlined in the preceding chapters. Therefore, this volume gives a foundation for the understanding of the companion volume, where the existing body of English-language literature is reviewed and classified. The aim is to illustrate the varying degrees of sophistication in approach among the existing studies. This should help the reader to interpret the results of each study with the appropriate amount of caution and to identify areas within his own field of interest where more analysis is required.

Major points from this chapter

1. Appraisal is concerned with the analysis of alternative courses of action with a view to assisting choice.

2. Because of the scarcity of resources, the criterion of economic efficiency is relevant when considering alternative strategies.

3. Cost = sacrifice (of the benefits to be derived from the use of a particular resource in its best alternative use).

4. Social costs and benefits (to the community) are merely the sums of the costs and benefits accruing to all individuals in the community.

5. Economists are not just interested in the effects of health services on national production.

6. Economic appraisal is a complement to, rather than a substitute for, medical appraisal. Assessment of medical effectiveness is normally an important preliminary stage in the assessment of efficiency.

7. In the provision of health care, many communities take into account considerations other than efficiency. These may be taken as constraints upon how far one might pursue efficiency, but do not deny the importance of efficiency as a criterion for appraising the provision of health services.

REFERENCES

Cochrane, A. L. (1972). *Effectiveness and efficiency—random reflections on health services*. Nuffield Provincial Hospitals Trust.
DHSS (Department of Health and Social Security) (1976a). *Sharing resources for health in England—Report of the resource allocation working party*. DHSS.
—— (1976b). *Priorities for health in England*. DHSS.
SHHD (Scottish Home and Health Department) (1976). *The health services in Scotland—the way ahead*. SHHD.
—— (1977). *Scottish Health Authorities revenue equalisation*. SHHD.

2

Costs and benefits in health care

Just what *is* involved in undertaking economic appraisals in the field of health care? This question is answered in detail in the chapters that follow. The purpose of this chapter is to give the reader an early glimpse of the economist's calculus. In particular, answers to the following questions will be sought: what are the relevant costs and benefits of health treatments; what is the cost–benefit approach? Figure 2.1 gives a schematic view of this chapter.

2.1. What are the relevant costs and benefits?

2.1.1. Costs

It will be remembered from Chapter 1 that the costs of a particular treatment are related to the resource sacrifices that it implies. Therefore, the economist is interested in the changes in resource use brought about by treatments. For most treatments, the majority of

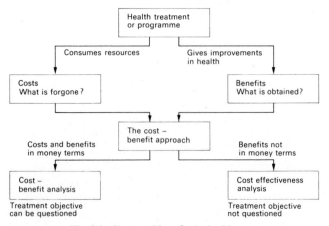

Fig. 2.1. Costs and benefits in health care.

these changes are likely to arise in the health care sector itself. For example, most treatments will require land, buildings, manpower, equipment, and consumable supplies. Note that the economist would not restrict consideration to resources for which money has to be paid. Those valuable resources that the organization already owns should not be ignored. Thus, just because no rental is charged for floor space, it should not be regarded as 'free' since, if it has an alternative use, its use in one treatment involves a sacrifice of the benefit that would be derived from using it in another. Also it should be noted that in economic terms it makes no sense to consider the resource consequences of a particular treatment in only *one* part of the health care sector. For example, a cost comparison of two treatments whose prime difference is in length of hospital in-patient stay should include consideration of the resource changes that shorter stays induce elsewhere in the health care system (e.g. increased demands upon community nursing services).

Of course many health treatments bring about resource changes in other sectors of the economy. In the UK context, the most obvious of these are the local authority resources used in health treatments, especially in the care of groups such as the elderly. Less obvious perhaps are the resources that patients and their families consume in obtaining treatment. For example, patients use up their own time in travelling to, or obtaining treatment at, health service facilities. In addition, relatives may have to spend time nursing patients confined at home. Sometimes the sacrifice made may be forgone leisure time; at other times patients and relatives may have to give up working time. Both working time and leisure time are valuable. Other important household resources consumed by health treatments include those used in self-medication, in transport to hospital or surgery, and in home adaptation. Often this resource usage will not involve the health service in expenditure, but in economic terms these changes still represent costs to the community, even though some of the resource usage in this category does not involve any cash transactions—e.g. housewives' time is not normally priced.

Just as not all costs involve money outlays so, conversely, not all cash transactions imply costs. An example here is the cash payments made to persons who are removed from the work-force through sickness. These payments are of importance, particularly to those who receive them and those government departments on whose budget they fall. Nevertheless they do not represent costs to the community as a whole since they do not involve resource usage.† They merely represent *transfers* of income or wealth from one section of the community to another, in this case a transfer from taxpayers to the sick.‡ These payments may well be significant from the equity viewpoint, but from the efficiency viewpoint the true cost to the community of the removal of a person from the work-force is the benefit to be derived from the use of that person's time in its best alternative use, in this case productive activity. Similarly, the tax revenue that the government receives when a sick person returns to work is not a net benefit of treatment, since it is merely a cash transfer from that individual to the community as a whole (of which he is a member). The community *as a whole* is no better or worse off if the tax is paid, though the distribution of net financial costs and benefits can, obviously, have implications from an equity standpoint, and may need to be estimated when that criterion is considered.

Therefore, in estimating the costs of treatments the economist will want to consider all the resource changes brought about by those treatments, irrespective of the sector of the economy in which these occur, and irrespective of whether the changes involve money outlays.§

2.1.2. Benefits

The most obvious effect of many health treatments is that the natural history of disease is changed for the better. That is, life may be extended, or the quality of life may be improved. This improvement may be the result of the removal of pain and suffering, or the result of improvements in mobility. All of these changes represent (economic) benefits since members of the community value good health *per se*. (A useful test of whether a change represents a benefit

---

† Some costs are involved, as resources are used in the administration of social security payment systems. However, the payments made are not estimates of these costs.

‡ In fact in many cases the sick person will be a taxpayer himself.

§ The investigation of the *financial* effects of treatment alternatives on government agencies may also be of importance. This analysis is properly termed a *public sector financial appraisal* and should not be confused with the form of economic appraisal known as *cost–benefit analysis*, which will be discussed below.

is whether the individual concerned would be willing to pay for the change. Most of us value good health enough to pay for it although in the UK the only sacrifice (cost) we are normally called upon to make it our own time and energy in obtaining treatment, or in maintaining a 'healthy' life-style. As noted in Chapter 1, one unfortunate feature of *practical* economic appraisal to date is that it has concentrated on measuring the benefits to be derived from just one aspect of 'being healthy': that is, the benefits, in increased production, of individuals being able to return to work.)

The benefits of health treatments are not confined to the individual whose health state is improved. Most of us derive benefit from the return to health of our relatives, friends and other individuals whom we may not even know. As far as possible, these benefits should be included in the assessment of total social benefit, but often they are likely to be omitted because of the cost of estimating them. (In any evaluative work one has to draw the line somewhere. In principle, this question is itself one for cost–benefit analysis—is the extra information worth the extra cost of obtaining it?). Returning to the question of return to work, a frequent benefit from a health treatment is that it enables *someone other* than the patient to resume employment.

Finally, some treatments, particularly preventive ones, may not have a perceptible effect on the patient's present health state, but may give him reassurance about his health *in the future*. For most people this reassurance would be worth paying for, and hence would count as a benefit.

2.2. The cost–benefit approach

It can be seen from the discussion above that in principle the economist takes a very wide view of the costs and benefits of health treatments. Correspondingly, the data requirements of an economic appraisal are likely to be greater than those of merely a financial or medical appraisal. Data will be required on the changes in resource use in all affected sectors and on the medical and social effects of treatment. In some cases, methods of valuing costs and benefits will have to be devised where no obvious valuations exist. The methods of assessing the costs and benefits of health treatments are dealt with in detail in Chapter 4. However, bearing in mind the difficulties involved, it may be worthwhile enquiring at this stage how the economist handles such a diverse set of information.

The techniques used can be encompassed under the general heading 'The cost–benefit approach'. First and foremost, the cost–benefit approach is a way of thinking. That is, it envisages *explicit* consideration on economic grounds, of the gains and losses associated with various courses of action. The two techniques under the cost–benefit umbrella are *cost–benefit analysis* and *cost effectiveness analysis*. The essential difference between the two is that in cost–benefit analysis an attempt is made to express *all* the costs and benefits outlined above in the same unit of account. The unit usually chosen is money.† As we shall see later, some categories of change brought about by health treatments are difficult to express in money terms and so the analysis will be incomplete. Here the decision maker will need to make a judgement of the valued items against the unvalued, and in so doing he is supplying, intuitively, the missing valuations. However, in all cases the analysis is best regarded as a useful aid to decision-making rather than as a substitute for it!

Alternatively, it is sometimes possible to assist choice by using the more limited variant—*cost effectiveness analysis*. This is appropriate when one is comparing two ways of meeting the same objective. If two alternative courses of action meet the objective equally well, then the less costly would be chosen on efficiency (or cost effectiveness) grounds. Of course, this approach is more restricted in that the worth of meeting the objective is not being questioned. Neither is one questioning the *extent* to which that objective should be met compared with others currently being considered. Nevertheless, the cost effectiveness approach does offer a number of methodological simplifications and the value of using it should not be underestimated. The instances where the cost effectiveness approach can be used are discussed more fully in Chapter 4.

Avid readers of the cost–benefit literature will notice that many authors do not follow the division of the consequences of health

---

† Money is chosen merely because it is a common unit for comparing the relative value of items. The use of money does not imply that economists feel that health services should 'make a profit'.

treatments (into 'costs' and 'benefits') adopted in §2.1. For instance, obviating the need to consume health care resources in the future through prevention can legitimately be viewed as a *benefit* of the preventive treatment. After all, these resources are being freed for alternative uses where they will generate benefits in terms of improved health. In the context of a given cost–benefit study the terms 'benefits' and 'costs' are often used as synonyms for the advantages and disadvantages respectively of particular courses of action. There is little wrong in this provided that the author of the study is consistent, but care is needed in practice. In the long run fewer misunderstandings are likely to be caused if the term 'benefit' is reserved for the 'improvements in health that various treatments or health programmes bring about'. There are two reasons for this. First, the use of the term 'benefit' for what are in essence 'cost off-sets' may lead the reader (and sometimes the author!) of a particular study to overlook certain important changes that treatments bring about. Preventive treatments again provide a good example. The real benefits from successful screening for, and fully effective earlier treatment of, a condition are measured by what people would be willing to pay in order to avoid any pain and discomfort (or more serious changes in health) associated with the progression of the condition in the absence of screening. The full magnitude of this saving is not captured merely by considering, say, future savings in medical resources.

Second, some of the decision indices discussed in Chapter 6 are sensitive to whether the particular effects of treatments are classed as costs or benefits. (See §6.2.2 for further discussion of this point.)

Major points from this chapter

1. The costs of health treatments do not all fall on the health service. They fall in addition, on patients, their families, and other public sector agencies.

2. Not all costs involve expenditure. Some resources are used (i.e. denied other uses) although no payment is made for their use.

3. Not all expenditure implies that a real resource cost to the community has been incurred.

4. The central benefit from health treatments is that they change the patient's health state (for the better). One (but only one)

dimension of this change is that the patient may be able to return to work and hence produce goods and services for the community.

5. The benefits from health treatments are not confined to the person receiving treatment.

6. For most choices in the field of health care, it is desirable to express all the relevant costs and benefits in commensurate units. This may not always be practicable and, either a more restricted question needs to be posed, or the decision-maker must exercise more of his own judgement.

7. It is best to think of the cost–benefit approach as a way of organizing thought rather than as a substitute for it.

3

Setting up an economic appraisal in health care

Most scientific work benefits from careful thought in the design stages, and economic appraisal is no exception. This is particularly important when one remembers the data requirements implicit in the outline of the economist's calculus given in Chapter 2. The purpose of this chapter is to give these important preliminaries a further airing before moving, in Chapter 4, to the detail of cost and benefit assessment. For a schematic view of this chapter see Fig. 3.1.

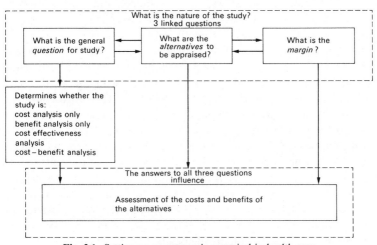

Fig. 3.1. Setting up an economic appraisal in health care.

3.1. Being clear on the study question

The questions tackled to date by economic appraisals can be summarized as follows:

1. What is the cost of treatment?
2. What is the benefit from treatment?

3. What is the most efficient way to treat a given condition?
4. Is the treatment worthwhile?

Of course the answers to questions (1) and (2) each provide only half the information required to arrive at a decision between alternative courses of action. A costly treatment should not be discontinued until the benefits it produces are estimated and compared with its costs. Similarly, the fact that a treatment is beneficial does not justify its instigation without a consideration of the cost at which those benefits are obtained. Nevertheless, studies dealing with only the cost or only the benefit of treatment have been important in the development of economic appraisal, because this restriction in scope has often enabled the analyst to break new ground in cost or benefit estimation. For this reason, studies of this type have been included in the review and classification of studies given in the companion volume. In particular the reader should note the studies by Wager (1972) and Dunnell and Ide (1974), both of which investigate those costs falling outside the health sector, on other public sector agencies or on patients and their families. On the benefit side, studies of particular note are those by Rosser and Watts (1972, 1974), who assess the relative value of particular defined health states, and by Jones-Lee (1976), who assesses the value to individuals of changes in the probability of their own death.

Studies designed to answer questions (3) and (4) must give explicit consideration both to costs and benefits. However, there is one important difference in study design between the two groups. In asking the question 'what is the most efficient way to treat a given condition' it is accepted that the condition will be treated. That is, it is automatically considered worthwhile to fulfil the treatment objective. As noted in Chapter 2, this simplifies the study design, and cost effectiveness analysis can be used. For example, if two treatments are found to be equally medically effective, then the changes in resource use brought about by them can be assessed and the least costly treatment preferred on economic grounds. This was the approach used by Piachaud and Weddell (1972) in their comparison of surgery with injection-compression sclerotherapy for the treatment of varicose veins, and Russell, Devlin, Fell, Glass, and Newell (1977) in their comparison of day-case surgery with traditional in-patient management for the treatment of inguinal herniae and haemorrhoids. In both the cases cited, the assumption of equal medical effect was tested through a randomized controlled trial.

The valuation of benefits can also be avoided where the treatments do not produce equivalent medical effects but where there is one clear objective of medical intervention and the 'success' of that intervention can unambiguously be measured. For example, if the objective of medical intervention in the case of a given disease were to prevent death, then alternatives could be compared on the basis of cost per year of life gained. (The logic here is that, for a given budget, the number of years of life gained would be greater if the more 'cost-effective' treatment were selected.) This was the approach used by Klarman, Francis, and Rosenthal (1968) in their comparison of the transplantation, hospital dialysis, and home dialysis alternatives for chronic renal failure. The authors argue that one feature of all three treatments is 'their capability for prolonging lives that otherwise would be cut short' and that 'it is no oversimplification to express their contributions in terms of the number of life-years gained by beneficiaries'. Thus the three treatments were compared in terms of their cost per life year gained.

Both these approaches have their problems. Can one often find two treatments which produce identical medical effects? For example, another study of the alternative treatments for varicose veins (Hobbs 1974) suggests that, on the basis of a six-year follow-up, the two treatments are not medically equivalent.† Similarly, is the objective of medical intervention often clear-cut or the 'success' of treatment easily measurable? In the study of chronic renal failure cited above, Klarman *et al.* recognize that the *quality* of a year of life gained by transplant may be higher than that of a year gained by dialysis.

It is clear, therefore, that extra sophistication in analysis may be required even when the treatment objective is not being questioned. This usually amounts to some kind of relative valuation of defined health states and will be discussed later (see Appendix 3). Nevertheless, the simplifications offered by cost effectiveness analysis are attractive and its use should always be considered.

---

† This result has recently been confirmed by a 5-year follow-up on Piachaud and Weddell's series of patients. It was found that 40 per cent of patients treated initially by injection/compression sclerotherapy were given further treatment, compared with 24.2 per cent of those treated initially by surgery (see Beresford *et al.* (1978)).

The question 'is the treatment worthwhile?' logically precedes the question of the most efficient way to treat. It is a question which is often taken for granted. In many situations this may be a reasonable course of action to take; there is hardly the need to question the worth of a highly effective and inexpensive drug therapy for an otherwise fatal disease. However, the worth of some treatments may be more open to question. If the treatment of patients required no sacrifices of scarce resources, then every medically effective treatment would be worthwhile. Since this is not the case, the worth of a treatment depends in part upon the alternative uses to which the resources it consumes can be put. This question can be posed at different levels of generality. At a specific level, one could ask whether a particular treatment objective is worthwhile fulfilling compared with other local objectives. At a more general level, one could consider that the resources consumed by the treatment could be redeployed in other sectors of the economy. It can be seen that more difficult choices are involved, perhaps in the allocation of resources between different health client groups, or even between the users of health services and the users of schools, roads, and other goods and services provided both in the public and private sectors of the economy. This suggests that more sophisticated appraisal is likely to be required. Several features of such an appraisal came to mind. First, it is necessary to compare all alternatives with the benchmark of 'doing nothing'. (The same principle is embodied in the use of control groups in medical trials.) Second, it is usually necessary to express the costs and benefits of the alternatives in a common unit of account. Hence the type of appraisal carried out is usually a full *cost–benefit analysis*, where all costs and benefits are measured in money terms. Third, the question of the *distribution* of costs and benefits between individuals in the community is likely to gain more prominence, since the beneficiaries of the proposed alternative courses of action may differ. (This contrasts with the comparison of two alternative ways of treating a defined treatment population.) The issue of the distribution of costs and benefits is always present to some extent in all economic appraisals. (For more discussion see Appendix 2.)

3.2. The importance of marginal analysis

Although the above classification of study questions is useful in assessing the need for varying degrees of sophistication in economic appraisal, it requires an additional ingredient to make it more relevant to the ways in which choices are made in the real world. This missing ingredient is the notion of *the margin*. If one considers the question 'is the treatment worthwhile?' it is apparent that the question more frequently asked is that of *'how much* treatment would be worthwhile?' Choices in health care are not normally couched in terms of whether or not one should devote any resources at all (say) to the care of the mentally handicapped; rather, they are couched in terms of whether, given the current mix of health care provision, one should devote more or less resources to the care of the mentally handicapped. In this situation it is the *incremental (or marginal)* costs and benefits of expansion or contraction of the programme that are relevant, not the total costs and benefits of the whole existing programme.

It can be seen that the question of 'how much treatment' is really a series of questions relating to whether each successive increase in treatment is worthwhile. Clinicians will, no doubt, be familiar with the question of 'how much treatment?' in the context of individual patient management. In the planning context, the question often presents itself in the form of how extensive a particular service should be. For example, should an effective screening programme be expanded from high risk groups alone to the whole population? Obviously the decision-maker should take note of the incremental benefits obtained and the incremental costs incurred. The total costs and benefits of the existing programme are often likely to be a poor guide to these.

The notion of the margin is also important when considering the other study questions listed above. The answer to the question 'what is the most efficient way to treat a given condition?' will depend upon the existing pattern of provision and the size of the expansion required. Suppose than on average the treatment of a particular condition is more efficient by day-case surgery (i.e. equivalent medical effectiveness is obtained at lower cost). However, if the day-case unit in a given locality is working to capacity, the treatment of (say) an extra ten cases per week may prove more costly by day-case surgery than by traditional in-patient management, if there is spare capacity in the latter. (In order to treat the cases on a day-case basis, it may be necessary to convert existing wards into a day-case unit or to build a new unit.)

When a given service is not operating at full capacity, the

incremental cost (per case) of treating a few more cases may be much less than the average cost of the cases currently being treated, since this average cost may contain an element of overheads which would not increase if a limited number of extra cases were added. For example, adding extra patients to a half-empty ward will not increase consumption of heating and lighting. Nevertheless, if the margin being considered were an extra 200 cases per week it might well be worth considering converting other hospital buildings into a day-case unit, or building a new unit.

Therefore, it is important to be clear on the *size* of the change being investigated as well as the nature of that change. Of course sometimes the margin being investigated will be the provision of a new service. Here the marginal costs will coincide with the total costs of providing the new service.

3.3. Statement of alternatives

Discussion of the notion of the margin highlights the need to be precise in the statement of the alternatives being appraised. The alternatives usually flow naturally from the study question; indeed the question for study will often be put to the analyst as a series of alternatives—'should we provide A or B?'. Since the existence of alternatives (i.e. room for manoeuvre) is an important prerequisite for appraisal, it is worthwhile discussing the nature of alternatives in health care and also whether in some situations no alternative (or only one course of action) exists.

Several broad types of alternative have been set out in Williams (1974). These include choices between different *places* of treatment (home versus institution), different *timing* of treatment (prevention versus cure later), different *illnesses*, and different *clients*. The setting of priorities between different illnesses and different clients is inherently more difficult, and indeed most examples of appraisal have been concerned with different modes of treatment for a given client group with a given condition or group of conditions. Actual specified treatment alternatives may embody more than one of these broad sets of alternatives. A preventive treatment, say, is likely to involve less institutionalization than a curative treatment. In fact most of the previous discussion (and that to follow) is concerned with defined alternative treatment regimens, each embodying various combinations of the broad alternatives. However, it must be remembered that there are other important choices in the provision of health care not specifically linked to treatment, such as the siting of health service facilities, that present opportunities for economic appraisal.

The explicit statement of alternatives is important since the economic analyst is relying on the imagination, ingenuity, and thoroughness of the health care specialist to specify the proper range of treatment alternatives for medical and economic appraisal. How do such alternatives arise? Very often treatment alternatives clearly present themselves—the obvious alternative to a new treatment is the one currently in common use. Occasionally, alternative treatments develop in parallel over a number of years.

In the context of planning services for groups of patients, the discussion of alternatives often raises problems. In particular, the following questions are often raised:

1. *Are not some 'alternative' regimens really complementary?* An example here is found in the treatments for chronic renal failure. Although long-term dialysis can be considered to be an alternative to transplantation, dialysis could also be considered to be a complement, in that patients are often dialysed prior to transplantation. In addition, many patients return to dialysis if the transplanted kidney fails. The way forward in this situation is to consider *combinations* of the dialysis and transplantation regimens. That is, the difficulty is overcome by recognizing that there are numerous combinations of the main treatment options, each constituting an 'alternative'. There are many other instances of combinations of treatments, such as drug therapy and radiotherapy in the management of patients with cancer.

2. *Is one ever faced with no alternative?* It should be clear by now that in any situation there is always the alternative of 'doing nothing'. Usually, those who argue that there is 'no alternative' but to treat a given condition mean that, in their judgement, the benefits from treatment far outweigh the costs. Even then there is the question of 'how much treatment', alluded to in §3.2. At each decision point the alternative is between further treatment and no more treatment, the relevant (economic) consideration being the comparison of the value of the expected benefit from the next block of treatment (if given) with its costs.

3.4. Some pitfalls for the unwary

The most obvious pitfall in setting up an appraisal is that of not matching the method of appraisal to the question being posed. It occurs in two guises:

1. *Failure to appraise the implicit alternative of 'doing nothing'.* If the intention is to ascertain whether treatment is worthwhile, then the alternative of 'doing nothing' requires explicit appraisal. Failure to do so has occasionally presented analysts with problems. For example, in interpreting the results of an appraisal of treatments for rheumatic diseases undertaken by Brooks (1971), we must assume that all the measured improvement (in terms of return to work by patients) was due to the treatments being given. This is because of the absence of a control group of patients for which the disease was allowed to take its course. This further emphasizes the attractions of linking economic appraisal to prospective clinical evaluation (as carried out in randomized controlled trials). Of course, there are situations where it is difficult to carry out such trials and here the possibilities for economic appraisal will be limited. Thus the case cited above is probably one in which many would argue that it would be unethical to withhold treatment in order to set up a control group.

2. *Exclusion of an important treatment alternative.* In a study of a five-bed coronary care unit in a district general hospital, Reynell and Reynell (1972) calculate the cost per life saved in the unit, suggesting that 'this kind of outcome analysis by survival could be used to assess the performance of other types of coronary care unit and other forms of expensive medical treatment'. While it is indeed important to find out the effectiveness of, say, coronary care units in saving lives, and to ascertain their running costs, the 'assessment of performance' of expensive medical treatments is best carried out by comparison with possible alternative therapies. In the case of coronary care units, relevant alternatives would include treatment in an ordinary hospital ward and treatment at home. Although Reynell and Reynell initially restricted their analysis to patients requiring resuscitation from cardiac arrest, the home care alternative could not be completely excluded from their study. This was because the very existence of the coronary care unit diverted patients from this alternative therapy.

Major points from this chapter

1. A number of questions can be answered by economic appraisal. Different questions require different levels of sophistication in analysis.

2. Choices between treatments require the consideration of both relative costs and relative benefits.

3. If the question of whether the treatment is worthwhile is being tackled, then the alternative of 'doing nothing' must be explicitly appraised.

4. If the question of whether the treatment is worthwhile is *not* being tackled, then the possibility exists for simplification in the analysis. (This more restricted approach is called *cost effectiveness analysis*.)

5. Usually, it is the *marginal* or incremental costs and benefits of expansion or contraction of a given programme that are relevant, not the total costs and benefits of the programme.

6. There is always more than one course of action. The existence of alternatives gives the scope for appraisal.

7. It is important to match the alternatives being appraised to the question being asked.

REFERENCES

Beresford, S. A. A. *et al.* (1978). Varicose veins: a comparison of surgery and injection compression sclerotherapy. *Lancet*, April 29, 921–4.
Brooks, R. (1969). A cost-benefit analysis of the treatment of rheumatic diseases. *Ann. Rheumat. Dis.*, **28**, 655–61.
Dunnell, K. and Ide, L. (1974). An attempt to assess the cost of home care. In *Impairment, disability and handicap* (ed. D. Lees and S. Shaw). Heinemann for SSRC, London.
Hobbs, J. T. (1974). Surgery and sclerotherapy in the treatment of varicose veins: a random trial. *Arch. Surg.*, **109**, 793–6.
Jones-Lee, M. W. (1976). *The value of life: an economic analysis*. Martin Robertson, London.
Klarman, H. E., Francis, J. O'S., and Rosenthal, G. D. (1968). Cost effectiveness analysis applied to the treatment of chronic renal disease. *Medical Care*, **6**, 48–54.
Piachaud, D. and Weddell, J. M. (1972). The economics of treating varicose veins. *Int. J. Epidemiol.*, **1** (3), 287–94.
Reynell, P. C. and Reynell, M. C. (1972), The cost-benefit analysis of a coronary care unit. *Brit. Heart J.*, **34**, 897–900.
Rosser, R. M. and Watts, V. C. (1972). The measurement of hospital output. *Int. J. Epidemiol.*, **1** (4), 361–8.

Rosser, R. M. and Watts, V. C. (1974). The development of a classification of the symptoms of sickness and its use to measure the output of a hospital. In *Impairment, disability and handicap* (ed. D. Lees and S. Shaw). Heinemann for SSRC, London.

Russell, I. T., Devlin, H. B., Fell, M., Glass, N. J., and Newell, D. J. (1977). Day case surgery for hernias and haemorrhoids: a clinical, social and economic evaluation. *Lancet*, **i**, 844–7.

Wager, R. (1972). *Care of the elderly—an exercise in cost benefit analysis commissioned by Essex County Council*. I.M.T.A. (now Chartered Institute of Public Finance and Accountancy), London.

Williams, A. H. (1974). The cost benefit approach. *Brit. med. Bull.*, **30** (3), 252–6.

4

Assessment of costs and benefits

The assessment of the costs and benefits of the alternative strategies being considered is the core of any economic appraisal. It is best to think of this assessment as consisting of three distinct stages. These are: *enumeration* of the relevant costs and benefits, *quantification (or measurement)* of the costs and benefits in physical units, *explicit valuation* of the costs and benefits in commensurate units. These stages are set out in Fig. 4.1 (see next page) and are discussed in turn below.

4.1. Enumeration of the relevant costs and benefits

At the beginning of a study it is essential to spend some time enumerating all those categories of cost and benefit that are considered important. This is just a listing, and should be considered separately from the quantification and valuation process. This is important since it ensures that the immeasurable changes brought about by health treatments remain as prominent as the measurable. In situations where some costs and benefits cannot be expressed in money terms, it is important that the decision-maker has a clear description of the unmeasured to consider in conjunction with the measured. (Making a decision inevitably involves a trade-off between the measured and the unmeasured.)

The relevant costs and benefits of health treatments were enumerated in Chapter 2. These can be classified as follows:

Changes in resource use;
Changes in productive output;
Changes in health state *per se*.

4.1.1. Changes in resource use

1. *Health service resources*: e.g. land, buildings, manpower, equipment, consumable supplies.

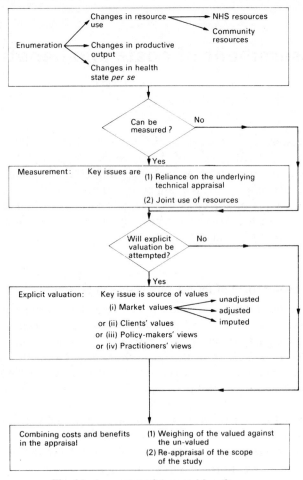

Fig. 4.1. Assessment of costs and benefits.

2. *Other support services* (*outside the health service*): local authority services (especially Social Services); voluntary services. (Note: although these are obtained 'for free' their use in one treatment would imply a cost if this prevented their use in another beneficial activity. However, voluntary resources are often given

for specific purposes only and would not necessarily be available to be used in other health programmes if no longer required in a particular treatment.)

   3. *Patients' (and their families') resources.*
   (*a*) *Personal time*: in being in hospital; in waiting at, or travelling to, health service facilities, for own treatment or the treatment of others; in being confined at home; in nursing patients confined at home.

Some of this time will be taken from work time, so the community may lose productive output (see below). However, some of the time may be taken merely from the patient's leisure time. Even leisure time has a value. (Would you prefer to be engaging in your favourite leisure pursuit, or to be waiting for a consultation, test, or treatment?) Often the distinction between leisure time and productive (work) time is blurred. Into which category does digging the vegetable garden fall? However, the principle is clear, the cost associated with the use of time is the value of that time in its best alternative use.

   (*b*) *Drugs and dressings provided by the household.*

   (*c*) *Transport.* Families often use their own resources in travelling to health service facilities.

   (*d*) *Home adaptation.* This is important, say, in the case of home dialysis. If a room in the house is turned over solely to dialysis, the family forgoes the value of that room in its alternative use. In addition, the family may need to commit resources in the adaptation of the home to accommodate, say, a disabled member of the family. (For examples of home adaptation costs see Buxton and West (1975), and Dunnell and Ide (1974)).

   (*e*) *Special diets.*

This list of the family's resource consumption is not meant to be exhaustive. Some conditions may involve patients or their families in extra expenditure on telephones, laundry, electricity, and so on.

Indeed, one could go to great lengths in itemizing all aspects of family expenditure. However, this can involve a great deal of time and expense, and the question of 'how far one should go?' is discussed later (in §4.4). Nevertheless, the example below should serve to illustrate the dangers of not considering patients' costs. Suppose one were comparing institutional and domiciliary care for the elderly. Should one include, as a cost of domiciliary care, the expenditure on food, heating, and lighting provided by the elderly patient or his or her family? After all, that person would have to eat and to heat and light their house in any case. The answer is 'yes' if one were trying to compare the cost of domiciliary support with the cost of institutional care, since the cost estimates of the latter typically include the cost of food, heating, and lighting. (For an expansion of this argument see Wager 1972.) Again, the economist's main interest is in whether the community *as a whole* consumes a resource, not *who* pays.

4.1.2. Changes in productive output

These effects are important to the community since production is a major wealth-creating activity. Health treatments can effect changes in productive output in both directions. One of the principal effects of many treatments is to remove disability or debility and so, as well as making the individual feel better in himself, enable him to resume productive activity. It may be that some clinicians already take note of this change, in giving a higher priority to patients whose condition is causing them to lose work time. Conversely, many treatments, through necessitating the temporary confinement of the individual at hospital or at home, may (if the individual were engaged in productive activity immediately before treatment) cause a reduction in productive output in the short run.

To those treating a patient, the most obvious effect of a loss of work time is the individual's loss of income, although this loss may be cushioned somewhat by social security payments. However, in an over-all efficiency study, it is the loss of the productive output to the community as a whole that is important. Therefore all the changes in productive output brought about by health treatments are relevant, irrespective of whether that output normally attracts a wage. Thus, loss of housewives' productive time (which is usually unpaid) is just as relevant as the loss of factory workers' productive time (although these may have different values). Appendix 6 discusses the use of earnings data in economic appraisals in health care.

4.1.3. Changes in health state per se

For most clinicians, changes in patients' health states are the most obvious effects of engaging in health treatments. The recovery of the ability to return to work (and hence produce) is *one* important dimension of the change in health state induced by many treatments, but it represents only *part* of the total value of the change produced. Therefore, changes in productive output are possibly best thought of as only a subset of the changes in health brought about by treatment, although they have been given a great deal of attention by economists in the past. The main reason for this was given in §2.1.2.

However, for many of the treatments given, the changes in productive output may be negligible, but these treatments may still be worthwhile since they bring about improvements in the welfare of the individuals concerned. Some of the (economically) relevant components of changes in health state are already noted as part of the medical assessment of the relative 'success' of treatments (e.g. fatality rates, complication rates, etc.) Since the aim of economic appraisal is to value these changes, its data requirements are likely to be more extensive. It may require more detailed assessment of the changes in social functioning experienced by patients during and after treatment; for instance, the levels of pain experienced, general mobility, and the ability to perform certain everyday tasks such as wash, dress, feed oneself. As well as constituting part of the (broadly defined) medical outcome of treatment, these effects are legitimately included in an economic assessment since they affect how patients *value* the relative benefit of alternative treatments.

Another feature of the economic assessment of changes in health state previously referred to is that the value derived from better health is not confined to the patient. His family, friends, and other compassionate individuals *whom he may not even know* may derive benefit too. Ideally their valuations of the changes in health state brought about by treatment should be included too. In fact for some treatments, such as the case of the mentally handicapped or the care of elderly persons with senile dementia, it may be the value placed *by others* upon the benefits of treatment that is a key component in determining how much care is given, since the patients themselves may not be in a position to assess the benefits from care. All the relevant changes identified above are set out schematically in Fig. 4.2.

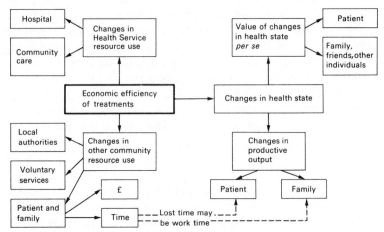

Fig. 4.2. The relevant changes in a comparison of the economic efficiency of treatments.

4.2. The measurement of costs and benefits

Once the relevant costs and benefits have been enumerated, the next stage is to measure the changes in these brought about by the treatments being appraised. For changes in resource use, the resource inputs to a treatment might be quantified in hours of nurses' time, hours of doctors' time, number of dressings, etc. Similarly, the changes in productive output brought about by a treatment could be quantified as the number of working days gained or lost. Usually, quantification is an important preliminary to valuation, i.e. it is necessary to know the size or number of gains and losses before they can be valued. Occasionally, difficulties in quantification may mean that it is easier to proceed to explicit valuation—this may be particularly true in the case of some of the changes in health state, where it is sometimes difficult to agree upon an unambiguous method of measurement. (For example, I might be able to give an estimate of what it would be worth to me for you to stop twisting my arm, although I might find it difficult to estimate whether the pain I am experiencing is twice or three times that which I experienced last week at the dentist's surgery!)

In particular, two issues in measurement will be stressed. These are the measurement of changes in health state, and the problems caused by the joint use of resources.

4.2.1. The measurement of changes in health state

An important component of the measurement of the change in health state brought about by treatment is the underlying medical appraisal. It was stressed earlier that economic appraisal is all the better for being based on thorough medical evaluation. It is not the intention here to become involved in the medical and statistical aspects of controlled clinical trials, other than to suggest that one is likely to be able to infer more from an economic appraisal based upon the results of a comprehensive, prospective clinical evaluation of specific treatments given to a defined patient population, than from one which has to draw upon piecemeal medical evidence from a variety of sources.

However, the economist does have an interest in how prospective evaluations are set up. On a practical level, he will be interested in whether facilities will exist for the collection of the data that he requires for his own evaluation work. (Hence it is beneficial to involve the economist at an early stage.) On a more fundamental level, the economist is likely to take an interest in the indicators used to assess the relative medical effectiveness (or 'success') of therapies. If the treatments remove patients' disabilities, he would be keen to see 'time taken to return to work' included as one measure of the success of treatment, since this information is vital to the assessment of changes in productive output. More generally, he would be interested in whether the indicators of medical effectiveness chosen are those in which the patient is likely to appreciate changes. 'Complication rates' are often used as a measure of the effectiveness of treatments. Are the 'complications' always those which a patient can appreciate? Is each 'complication' of equal disbenefit to the patient?

Of course, for many treatments the answer to the question of 'what to measure' is self-evident. Thus, for a life-saving treatment, the extension of life gained is an objective measure of 'success', although even then the 'quality' of the years gained is crucial. Schneiderman and Krant (1966) have suggested that in some branches of medicine the question of 'what to measure' is more open to debate:

> In a comparison of drugs, a higher objective response rate from a specific drug was not related to longer survival of the total number of patients receiving that drug, bringing the specific objective response (tumor measures) in these diseases into question. It is suggested that this objective response criterion does not measure the whole patient and may therefore be misleading.

These questions, of 'what to measure' and 'how to measure it', have become an area of common concern both to medical researchers and to economists and operational researchers. The economist's interest stems from the need to define 'states of health' in which changes can be appreciated by the sick person (or any other individual caring about that person's health). What has emerged is that several important value judgements are implicit in measuring changes in health. (These are discussed in Appendix 3.) However, it is clear that since the estimation of the medical effectiveness of treatments is crucial to the economic appraisal, the economist would want to participate in the design of a medical trial, in the same way as any statistician who is to analyse the results.

4.2.2. Joint use of resources

A major problem in the assessment of the changes in resource use brought about by treatments is that many resources are used *jointly* with our treatments. The problem is most apparent in the hospital where many of the resources, such as those used in heating and lighting, are used for the common good of all the patients in the hospital at a particular time. Some resources, such as nursing time, are partly consumed jointly and partly consumed on a personal basis. Thus a particular patient may enjoy individual nursing attention, but shares with other patients in the benefits derived from general nursing vigilance in the ward. How does one apportion such *joint costs* to particular patients, or to particular treatments? At first sight it looks as though one could have an infinite number of schemes for apportionment, depending upon the assumptions one is prepared to make. This is certainly one of the main conclusions which could be drawn from major studies in this area (see for instance, Babson 1973, Russell 1974). However, for planning purposes the problem is often simplified. Remembering the notion of *the margin* discussed in Chapter 3, it is only the *incremental or marginal* costs that are of relevance. That is, what are the *changes* in resource use brought about by the treatment alternatives being considered. This approach is likely to give a different answer from an *ad hoc* apportionment of existing costs. An application of this approach is contained in the work of Russell, Devlin, Fell, Glass, and Newell (1977). In a comparison of day-case surgery with traditional in-patient management, it was estimated that the instigation of day-case surgery for the conditions in question would, with given workloads, mean that either a small ward could be closed or that the construction of a small extension could be avoided. Both these represent situations where scarce resources could be freed for other uses—such as the treatment of more patients. (This example is discussed in more detail in Chapter 7.)

Often, it may not be possible to be so precise, particularly if one is trying to make estimates of resource savings nation-wide. Nevertheless, the principle should always be adhered to: in considering the proposed change, the key question is what extra resources would be required (or alternatively, what resources would be freed for other uses).

4.3. The explicit valuation of costs and benefits

This is the stage in the appraisal where values are placed on the various costs and benefits in order to render them commensurate with one another. It is also the stage in the appraisal which raises the most doubts in many peoples' minds, primarily because of its explicit use of value judgements. Discussion of value judgements raises questions about the 'objectivity' of the cost–benefit approach. These fears are understandable, particularly when one considers the difficult area of valuing the changes in health state brought about by health treatments. However, it is important to note that many of us may commit ourselves to certain value judgements unknowingly. For instance, many would accept market prices as representing true valuations of the resources used in health treatments. However, market prices are not value-free: they derive from a particular distribution of income and from a set of institutional and legal arrangements which allow trade in the commodities concerned. Also, planning decisions in health care will often imply valuations, say, of health improvement, although the valuation problem may not be faced explicitly. For instance, one can infer a valuation of life from the amount we, as a community, are willing to spend on life-saving programmes. In short, one cannot make public policy decisions without making value judgements of one sort or another.†

Various approaches to the valuation problem in health care are set out below. It is not the intention here to argue that one method is 'better' or 'more correct' than another since that would imply arguing for the superiority of one set of value judgements over another. However, it will be argued that it is better to make value judgements *explicit*.

4.3.1. Approaches to valuation

The traditional economics approach views the community as, and only as, a collection of individuals. The relevant valuations are those that these individuals make about factors concerning their own welfare. (This is not necessarily to imply a selfish attitude on the part of individuals, since included in one person's valuation are his feelings about the welfare of others). Individuals' valuations are reflected in *what they would be willing to pay*‡ to receive benefits or avoid costs. This approach has some important underlying value judgements. First, individuals are taken to be the best judges of their own welfare. Second, the existing distribution of income or wealth is accepted, since individuals' willingness to pay will be conditioned by their ability to pay. Not all the observed approaches to valuation embody these principles, possibly because some analysts fail to subscribe to these underlying value judgements, but possibly also because it is sometimes very difficult to make good direct estimates of willingness to pay. This is especially true of the changes in health state brought about by treatment. (It is worth noting that this is in part a product of the institutional arrangements for the provision of health care in the UK. Since individuals

---

† In addition, it is worth noting that measurement is not value-free. For instance, the medical researcher has scope for the exercise of judgement as to: how outcome is assessed; the method of allocation of subjects to treatment groups; the level of statistical significance to accept; and so on.

‡ Where 'pay' in this context is taken as a general measure of what people are willing to forgo (or sacrifice), rather than just the money amount.

are not often called upon to pay, other than in terms of the time and energy used to obtain treatment, no data on willingness to pay are generated.)

Market-based valuations. Of course if a market did exist for the 'products' of the health care system, then data on willingness to pay would be revealed and could be used as a basis for valuing the benefits of treatment. Even then, a complication would exist when taking the market price as an estimate of the willingness to pay for the commodity in question. If a single price prevails in the market place (as is often the case) the price paid by most consumers would *understate* their true willingness to pay. Only for those consumers who think that the item is 'just about worth buying at the price' will the price paid equal willingness to pay. Some consumers would have been prepared to pay more but, because the same price applies to everyone, they are not called upon to do so.

Turning to the valuation of the costs of treatments, markets do exist for most of the *resources* used in health treatments and market prices are the most common source of valuation. Thus,

The value of one hour of nurse's time = hourly wage rate (including associated employment costs);
The value of drugs and dressings = price paid for them

Thus, it can be seen that the economic and financial estimate of 'cost' will sometimes coincide.

However, how does the use of market prices relate to the economist's notion of cost outlined in Chapter 1, where the cost of a unit of a resource was defined as the benefit that would be derived from using it in its best alternative use? Although at the local level, the cost of, say, unnecessarily lengthening in-patient stays can be identified in terms of the benefits foregone in using those bed-days for the treatment of other patients, on a more general level market prices relate to what is foregone in the following way. In order to secure the resources for our own use (say, in a health treatment) we have to compete with other potential users, and we shall only obtain the required resources if we are prepared to pay at least what others were willing to pay for the use of them. Thus what we finish up paying will be a reflection of each resource's value in its best alternative use.

For market prices to reflect the 'true' value of commodities we have to assume that: consumers know what they are doing; markets are free of monopolistic elements; prices are not seriously 'distorted' by taxes and subsidies; there are no benefits accruing to, or costs falling on (non-participating) third parties as the result of market transactions. (Thus, if a person is vaccinated against a communicable disease he may also confer benefits, in the form of increased protection, on others who are not vaccinated. *Their* valuations of *his* vaccination will not be incorporated into the market price.)

Indeed there are further complexities which cannot be discussed here, but it suffices to say that, subject to the qualifications outlined above, market prices (where they exist) may give the economist reliable estimates of the values he seeks to obtain. However, on a practical note, market prices tend to be used more often than not because they are readily available.

So far the use of market prices in their *unadjusted* form has been mentioned. Two variations on this are discussed below.

1. *Adjusted market prices.* Sometimes adjustments are made to 'correct' market prices where market imperfections, such as monopolistic elements or taxes and subsidies, exist. For example, Wager (1972) regarded fuel prices are overstating the true value (in opportunity cost terms) of that resource, because of the imposition of high taxes. Since fuel cost was an important component of home nursing costs, he felt that home care had been made 'artificially expensive' relative to institutional care. Therefore, he deducted the fuel tax from his estimate of the cost of home nursing.

There are few other examples. The decision whether to adjust depends upon:

(a) The importance of the item itself in the over-all appraisal;
(b) The extent to which its market price seems likely to deviate from its 'true' value;
(c) The time and trouble (hence cost) of obtaining and processing the information needed to make the adjustments.

2. *Imputed market prices.* Although market prices may be useful for valuing some of the effects of health treatments, for many they do not exist at all. In these cases economists have sometimes tried to *impute* valuations, using associated market prices as a guide. For example:

Value of housewives' production. Here no wage is paid so we have no direct market price (earnings) as an estimate of the value of the production. However, some economists have used the wages of domestic helps as a basis for estimating the value of housekeeping production (e.g. Brooks 1969).

Patients' personal (i.e. non-working) time. We do not have a direct market price for this time but we observe that individuals do often trade time for money (say) through their purchase of quicker forms of travel, e.g. air instead of rail, underground instead of bus. Beesley (1965) calculated the value of time which best explained observed modal choices (between private car and public transport) of a sample of employees at the Ministry of Transport in London.

'Unpleasantness' of a particular illness. In his estimate of the costs of venereal disease, Klarman (1965) used patients' expenditures on medications (to alleviate a skin complaint, psoriasis) as an estimate of the unpleasantness associated with VD.

Obviously, imputed market valuations can only be as good as the closeness of fit between the 'proxy' and the 'target' situation. This has two aspects:

(a) Do people perceive these transactions in the same way as the market transactions that are to be approximated, and hence is their behaviour a good guide?

(b) Can one find an analogous market for the commodity in question, e.g. domestic help is not the only service housewives perform; in trading-off time one is also trading-off other amenities—do not some people prefer air travel *per se*; was Klarman's 'analogous' disease really similar enough to VD?

Non-market valuations. The use of market-based valuations accords closely with the traditional economic postulates set out at the beginning of §4.3.1. However, absence of market prices has caused economists to look for other sources of valuation. More fundamentally, it may be that in rejecting the idea of a market for health care many communities have indicated that they do not concur with the set of value judgements upon which market valuations are based. A number of alternative approaches to valuation have been used.

1. *Clients' views.* In the absence of adequate markets, analysts

have sometimes approached consumers directly for their valuations. This approach has been used mostly in connection with the valuation of changes in state of health. The methods used are variants of the simple question 'what would you be willing to pay?' for a stated improvement in state of health. However, the methods employed are very sophisticated and require more discussion than could be afforded in this guide. (Further reading is indicated in Appendix 3.)

An example of this approach is the study undertaken by Jones-Lee (1976), who estimated the amount that individuals were willing to pay for a reduction in the probability of their own death, by presenting them (through a questionnaire) with hypothetical situations where reductions in the probability of death were to be traded against extra money outlays. (The actual examples related airline fares to airline crash records, and health hazards from environmental pollution to house valuations.)

The main critics of these methods point to their (inevitable) hypothetical nature, hence the danger that respondents will (deliberately or inadvertently) give inaccurate answers.

2. *Policy-makers' views.* It has been suggested by some that policy-makers' views represent a legitimate source of values. One could take the view that if clients' preferences cannot be elicited, then perhaps these are mirrored by those whose job it is to make decisions that affect clients, especially if policy-makers are answerable in some way to the community. Alternatively, it might be argued that policy-makers are better judges of clients' welfare than clients themselves, because they are better informed of the many complex issues involved.

Values may be taken either from *explicit* statements by policy-makers, or inferred *implicitly* from their actions. Thus, the value of life has been *explicitly* stated as an entry in some cost–benefit appraisals of road improvements undertaken by the (UK) Department of the Environment.† Alternatively, the value of life

---

† It should be pointed out that this value was in turn estimated mainly by use of market-based valuations. The approach used was to consider the value of the net production loss through the death of an individual (estimated from average earnings). To this was added an amount reflecting the value of life *per se* (see Dawson 1971).

can be inferred *implicitly* from the value of the resources required to put into effect various forms of safety legislation.

The use of policy-makers' views is not without its practical problems—one feature of *implied* values is that they vary so greatly. However, the major objection to their use is that they often arise from the very kind of *ad hoc*, non-systematic decision-making process that economic appraisal is employed to improve.

3. *Practitioners' views (or professional opinion)*. Three sources of professional values can be identified in the existing literature; namely: the medical researcher or economic analyst; the health service professional; the courts. Again, these values may have been used by analysts for a variety of reasons: because of practical considerations; because there may be situations where the client is assumed *not* to be the best judge of his own welfare; or because the values generated will be independent of the prevailing income distribution (although some court awards may be based partly on the income of the injured party).

Examples of the use of practitioners' views can be found in the following studies by: Klarman, Francis, and Rosenthal (1968), who included a (researcher's) judgement that one year of life on dialysis was equivalent to 0.75 years with kidney transplant; Torrance, Sackett, and Thomas (1973) and Bush, Chen, and Patrick (1973) who used the values of physicians in deriving relative valuations of the desirability of various health states; Rosser and Watts (1972, 1974) who used court awards to derive relative valuations of the desirability of various health states.

4.3.2. Some issues in explicit valuation

The discussion of methods of explicit valuation often provokes one or other of the following reactions:

1. There are some effects which 'we just cannot value'.
2. Market prices are a 'superior' source of values.

Both of these arise out of genuine worries about the methods of explicit valuation used by economists. At the risk of repetition of some of the earlier arguments, they are discussed below.

1. *Are there some effects which 'we just cannot value'?* This claim is typically made of the outputs of health treatments; e.g. the

preservation of life, the removal of pain and disability, etc. Of course, the main implication of such a claim is that the community as a whole, or as individuals, would not know what proportion of its resources to devote to those activities (including health treatments) producing these effects. Since these decisions *are* made, it is clear that in fact these effects have been valued, albeit implicitly. (This is the basis for some of the methods of valuation outlined above.) In my view the debate is not really about whether or not these effects *can* be valued, but about the *source of values* and whether or not it should be *made explicit*. Deciding upon the proper source of values is not an issue which can be resolved by technical argument, since it involves arguing for the superiority of one set of value judgements over another. By contrast, a strong case can be made for explicit valuation processes on the grounds that they are more likely to lead to consistency in decision-making, and hence to better performance irrespective of the set of values held. For instance, a calculation of the value of life implied by willingness to accept the costs of implementing various kinds of safety legislation shows that these values vary markedly (see Mooney 1977).

If, as a community, we valued the lives saved by each safety programme equally, it would be more efficient to allocate resources so that the *incremental cost* of saving the last life by each method was the same. In a situation where this is *not* the case, then total resources could be re-allocated so as to save more lives in total. Of course, matters may not be that simple—the value of a life saved may depend on the age of the person† and the quality of that life. In addition, different ways of dying may have different degrees of unpleasantness attached to them.‡ However, the allocation of resources between life-saving programmes can only be brought into question if the implied values of saving life are revealed. Thus, why is it that in the UK we are willing to spend an average of £20 000 000 per life saved in prevention of a repetition of the Ronan Point Disaster,§ when we are not willing to spend anywhere near this

† Hence, 'years of life saved' is a better measure of the benefit obtained than 'lives saved'.

‡ Mooney (1977) gives a tentative list of the relevant factors in deciding upon these differentials. These include: age, family circumstances, the nature of the threat to life, the future expectation of life, the quality of future life and the 'fairness' of risk (i.e. is it self-imposed or not). Obviously, all these issues merit further discussion.

§ This was the collapse of a high-rise building in London.

amount per life saved in the kidney dialysis and transplantation programme? In addition, greater explicitness can help policy-makers decide whether enough *in total* is being spent on life-saving programmes.

2. *Are market prices a 'superior' source of values?* Of all the methods of explicit valuation outlined above, those involving market prices are the most widely accepted. Indeed, the market price is virtually the only source of values used in financial appraisal. Economists are often criticized for including in cost–benefit analyses the valuations of effects, such as time savings, not derived directly from observed market exchanges (see, in particular, Self 1970, 1975.) It is true that the main strength of market prices as a source of values is that they are the *observable* results of many individuals' behaviour. In that respect they probably represent 'harder' data than that typically obtained from presenting a few individuals with hypothetical situations. However, it must be re-membered that market prices are not value-free; they derive not only from the existing distribution of income, but also from the distribution of the time and energy and knowledge required to make market transactions; their use implies acceptance of the view that consumers are the best judges of their own welfare. In addition they may be subject to known imperfections such as those arising from the existence of monopoly power. Any one of these features may render them inappropriate in a particular context, so they cannot be regarded as a panacea for valuation problems.†

4.4. Combining costs and benefits in the appraisal

In outlining the various methods of explicit valuation above, the impression may have been given that the economist typically will want to measure and value *all* the changes brought about by the treatment alternatives in question. Although *in principle* he may want to do this, *in practice* it is not always the case that all the valuation questions are confronted 'head-on', nor that the widest possible range of factors is considered. For example:

1. If there is no intention to question whether or not treatment is worthwhile *per se*, the cost effectiveness approach can be used. In its simplest form, this avoids the difficult problem of valuing

† See Williams (1972) for a forceful reply to some of Self's criticisms.

changes in health state. (Remember that the two simple applications of the approach are (a) where the treatments produce
identical outcomes and (b) where there is one main objective of
treatment and the success in attaining this objective can be
measured.) The cost effectiveness approach can be applied in a
slightly more sophisticated form even in situations where neither of
these conditions is met. Here, the changes in health state brought
about by treatment are not valued in money terms, but are valued
relative to one another (see Appendix 3).

2. Some of the changes brought about by two alternatives may
be identical. Therefore, in answering the question 'what is the most
efficient way to treat?' only the *differences*, say, in the resource use
brought about by treatments need be costed. (In the hospital
setting, this could reduce considerably the analytical work
involved.)

3. Some of the changes most difficult to measure or value may
just reinforce the conclusions to be drawn from the changes which
can be valued. For example, if a preventive programme used less
resources than a curative programme, then the avoidance of any
pain, suffering, or discomfort associated with the latter would serve
to reinforce the view that the preventive programme should be
chosen.

4. Often the economist may not attempt to value changes in
health state but will present these for consideration alongside the
resource outlays. In a situation where the more costly alternative is
also the more effective, the decision-maker can then see the cost at
which greater effectiveness is being obtained. He can then consider
this option against other possible beneficial uses for those extra
resources used in the more costly alternative.

5. Finally, there are no limits to the extent of economic
information one could glean in order to inform decisions. In this
book the principles guiding the gathering of that information have
been set out, although the question 'how far should one go?' has
not been explicitly tackled. Of course, the now familiar arguments
ought to apply. Are the benefits (in terms of 'better' decisions)
greater than the costs? Obviously there will be situations where it
would not be worthwhile undertaking an economic appraisal, in the
same way that there are situations where it would not be

worthwhile to give more treatment. In these situations the economist's approach may be more usefully employed as *a way of thinking*, rather than as prescription for carrying out analytical work. However, there are many situations where economic appraisal is likely to be worthwhile. Williams (1974) provides a useful checklist.

Cost–benefit studies are most likely to pay off in situations where:

Sizeable amounts of scarce resources are at stake;
Responsibility is fragmented;
The objectives of the respective parties are at variance or unclear;
There exist alternatives of a radically different kind;
The technology underlying each alternative is well understood;
The results of the analysis are not wanted in an impossibly short time.

Major points from this chapter

1. There are *three* stages in the assessment of costs and benefits: enumeration, measurement, and explicit valuation.

2. The relevant changes brought about by health treatments are: changes in resource use, changes in productive output, changes in health state *per se*.

3. Economic appraisal relies partly on medical appraisal for the assessment of changes in health state. Therefore economic appraisal can only be as good as the medical appraisal upon which it is superimposed.

4. The major measurement problems in changes in resource use arise from the joint use of resources. This needs to be given careful consideration.

5. For the explicit valuation of the changes, there are a number of sources of value judgements, the use of each of which has its own rationale.

6. One cannot escape making value judgements in this area. The real question is whether these judgements are made explicit or not.

7. Although the data requirements of a full economic appraisal are potentially very extensive, a number of simplifications exist which can reduce the amount of work necessary.

REFERENCES

Babson, J. H. (1973). *Disease costing*. Studies in Social Administration, University of Manchester.

Beesley, M. E. (1965). The value of time spent in travelling: some new evidence. *Economica*, May, 174–85.

Brooks, R. (1969). A cost-benefit analysis of the treatment of rheumatic diseases. *Ann. Rheumat. Dis.*, **28**, 655–61.

Bush, J. W., Chen, M. M., and Patrick, D. L. (1973). Health status index in cost effectiveness: analysis of a P.K.U. program. In *Health status indexes* (ed. R. L. Berg). Hospital Research and Educational Trust, Chicago.

Buxton, M. J. and West, R. R. (1975). Cost benefit analysis of long term haemodialysis for chronic renal failure. *Brit. med. J.*, ii, pp. 376–9.

Dawson, R. F. F. (1971). Current cost of road accidents in Great Britain. *Ministry of Transport RRL Report LR79*. Road Research Laboratory, Crowthorne.

Dunnell, K. and Ide, L. (1974). An attempt to assess the cost of home care. In *Impairment, disability and handicap* (ed. D. Lees and S. Shaw). Heinemann for SSRC, London.

Jones-Lee, M. W. (1976). *The value of life: an economic analysis*. Martin Robertson, London.

Klarman, H. E. (1965). Syphilis control programs. In *Measuring benefits of government investments* (ed. R. Dorfman). Brookings Institution, Washington, DC.

——, Francis, J. O'S., and Rosenthal, G. D. (1968). Cost effectiveness analysis applied to the treatment of chronic renal disease. *Med. Care*, **6**, 48–54.

Mooney, G. H. (1977). *The valuation of human life*. Macmillan, London.

Rosser, R. M. and Watts, V. C. (1972). The measurement of hospital output. *Int. J. Epidemiol.* **1** (4), 361–8.

——, —— (1974). The development of a classification of the symptoms of sickness and its use to measure the output of a hospital. In *Impairment, disability and handicap* (ed. D. Lees and S. Shaw). Heinemann for SSRC, London.

Russell, E. M. (1974). *Patient costing study*. Scottish Health Services Studies No. 31, Scottish Home and Health Department.

Russell, I. T., Devlin, H. B., Fell, M., Glass, N. J., and Newell, D. J. (1977). Day case surgery for hernias and haemorrhoids; a clinical social and economic evaluation. *Lancet*, i, 844–7.

Self, P. (1970). Nonsense on stilts: cost-benefit analysis and the Roskill Commission. *Political Quart.*, **41** (3), 249–60.

—— (1975). *Econocrats and the policy process—the politics and philosophy of cost-benefit analysis*. Macmillan, London.

Schneiderman, M. A. and Krant, M. J. (1966). What shall we measure on whom: why? *Cancer Chemotherapy Rep.* **50** (3), 107–12.

Torrance, G. W., Sackett, D. L., and Thomas, W. H. (1973). Utility maximisation model for program evaluation: a demonstration application. In *Health status indexes* (ed. R. L. Berg). Hospital Research and Educational Trust, Chicago.

Wager, R. (1972). *Care of the elderly—an exercise in cost benefit analysis commissioned by Essex County Council*. I.M.T.A. (now Chartered Institute of Public Finance and Accountancy), London.

Williams, A. H. (1972). Cost–benefit analysis: bastard science? and/or insidious poison in the body politick. *J. public Econ.*, **1** (2), 199–225.

—— (1974). The cost benefit approach. *Brit. med. Bull.* **30** (3), 252–6.

5
Two refinements

The assessment of costs and benefits is the major component of any economic appraisal. However, there are two important refinements to this assessment procedure. These are: the allowance for the differential timing of costs and benefits; and, the allowance for risk and uncertainty in costs and benefits. See Fig. 5.1 for a schematic view of this chapter.

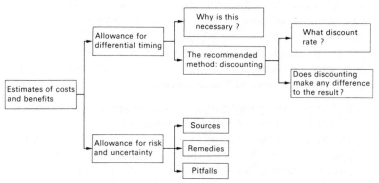

Fig. 5.1. A schematic view of Chapter 5.

5.1. Allowance for the differential timing of costs and benefits

The effects of health treatments do not all occur at the same point in time. Usually, the beneficial effects of therapy last not only for this year but also into the future. Similarly, some treatments demand continuing therapy and will require resources to be committed over a period of years, possibly for the patient's lifetime. Differences in the timing of costs and benefits are most obvious in the comparison of preventive treatments with their main alternative (treatment at the symptomatic stage). The preventive regimen requires that resources be committed at an earlier stage, in the expectation that those costs arising from the development of the condition at a later stage will be avoided. Setting aside for the moment some of the possible benefits of preventive treatment†, should one not differentiate between £1 spent now and £1 spent, say, in ten years time?

An answer to the above question can be found by observing how members of the community behave as individuals. When lending money to others we normally expect the borrower to pay a premium (i.e. interest). Typically we would demand the premium even in situations where we were certain to get the money back— where there is some risk attached to the enterprise, or where there is inflation, we might demand a higher premium. The reason for the premium is that, in lending the money to others, the individual would have to postpone some of his own spending until the time when the money is returned. Since most of us would prefer not to do that, we demand the premium as compensation. In economists' language, we are said to have a *positive* (*marginal*) *rate of time preference*.

Having established the existence of a positive rate of time preference, at least for members of the community acting as individuals, one must still decide upon:

1. The method of incorporating this concept into the appraisal of alternative courses of action in health care.‡
2. The appropriate rate of time preference to be assumed in the appraisal of public sector projects, since these really involve members of the community acting *collectively*, rather than as individuals.

The most widely accepted method of incorporating the time preference notion into the appraisal is the process of *discounting* costs and benefits arising in the future to equivalent *present values*. This amounts to multiplying the value of costs and benefits occurring in future years by a weighting factor, so that they can be compared as if they all occurred at the same point in time. The weights for each future year are derived with reference to the assumed rate of time preference, as follows:

---

† For example, the avoidance of the pain and suffering which may be present at the symptomatic stage, or the reassurance that preventive treatment may give.

‡ In this chapter, alternative courses of action will be referred to as 'projects'.

The existence of, say, a 10 per cent market rate of interest would suggest that lenders are indifferent (at the margin) between £100 now and £110 in one year's time. In algebraic terms:

If r = the annual rate of interest (0.1 in this case)
A = the amount this year in £s (£100 in this case)
B = the amount required after 1 year in £s

$B = A(1 + r)$,   i.e. £110

Generalizing to more than one year:

If C = the amount required after 2 years in £s

$$C = B(1 + r)$$
$$= A(1 + r)(1 + r)$$
$$C = A(1 + r)^2, \quad \text{i.e. £121.}$$

Therefore, it can be seen that after n years the amount required will be $A(1 + r)^n$. Discounting is just this compound interest calculation performed in reverse. Here we ask: 'what would one accept *now* instead of £110 in one year's time when the rate of interest is 10 per cent?' The answer is of course £100, and £100 is said to be the *present value* of £110 next year. In algebraic terms:

If B = an amount occurring in one year's time,
r = the rate of interest,
A = present value of B,

$$A = \frac{B}{1 + r}.$$

Similarly,

If C = an amount occurring in two years' time,
A = present value of C,

$$A = \frac{C}{(1 + r)^2}.$$

Therefore, it can be seen that the weights for 1, 2, and n years into the future are $1/(1 + r)$, $1/(1 + r)^2$, and $1/(1 + r)^n$, respectively. These are known as *discounting factors*, while r is known as the *discount rate*. Assuming a positive value for r, costs and benefits occurring in the future are multiplied by a factor less than unity, this factor becoming smaller as one moves more into the future. In practice, the calculation of the present values of costs and benefits is much simpler than it would appear at first sight since these factors (or weights) can be obtained from tables. Also, a worked example is given in Appendix 4.

The question of the appropriate public sector discount rate has been debated at some length by economists. It is possible only to give a brief outline of the debate in this text (in Appendix 4), but the practical question of choice of rate is often very easy to answer. In the UK for example, the Treasury recommends a rate for use throughout the public sector (this was 8 per cent in 1967, subsequently raised to 10 per cent in 1969, and then lowered to 7 per cent in 1977).

5.1.1. Does discounting, or the choice of discount rate, make much difference to the final result?

Discounting costs and benefits can make quite a difference to the final result, particularly if the alternative treatments being appraised vary greatly in the timing of their costs and benefits. A low discount rate is more likely to lead to the selection of a long-lived project, with net benefits occurring some distance into the future.

The importance of the choice of discount rate was shown by Cohn (1972) in his consideration of the 'eradication' and 'control' alternatives for malaria. 'Eradication' involves committing more resources earlier, in the expectation that once the condition is virtually eradicated (complete eradication being impossible) only

TABLE 5.1 *Present value of the costs of malaria control and eradication (in millions of rupees)*

Discount rate (per cent)	Control (for 30 years)	Eradication
6	930	654
8	761	613
10	636	574
12	545	542
14	473	508
16	417	479

Source: Cohn (1972).

minimal resources will be required. By contrast, the 'control' alternative requires a steady commitment of resources over the years. It can be seen from Table 5.1 that at lower discount rates the 'eradication' alternative is to be preferred on cost grounds. (We will assume for the moment that the two programmes are equivalent in respect of benefits.) However, as the discount rate is increased, the outlays in future years are given progressively less weight. This affects the 'control' alternative mostly, since 'eradication' does not involve many resource outlays in the future. At a discount rate of 12 per cent the present value of the costs is approximately the same, but at discount rates above 12 per cent the 'control' alternative would be preferred on cost grounds.†

5.1.2. Is discounting ever unnecessary?

Discounting would be unnecessary if:

1. Our rate of time preference were equal to zero; or
2. All the effects brought about by the health treatments under appraisal occurred over a period so short that the relative timing of costs and benefits did not matter; or
3. One project completely 'dominated' the other (i.e. the net benefits being greater in each and every year).

Condition (1) is unlikely to be met, but it is sometimes possible to arrange the study in order to satisfy condition (2). Suppose one were comparing day-case surgery with traditional in-patient surgery for a condition such as inguinal hernia. In addition, suppose that the medical effectiveness of the two treatments were identical and therefore our main concern was with relative cost. Here the resource usage associated with either treatment is likely to spread only over a matter of weeks or months and discounting would not

---

† The discerning reader will have noted that Cohn considered the costs for the first 30 years only. What about the costs after 30 years, one might ask? True, control will still involve sizeable resource outlays, whereas the outlays in maintaining the eradication programme are likely to be minimal. However, the discounting procedure is only reflecting the underlying assumption of a positive rate of time preference. For example, an outlay of £100 occurring in 30 years time has a present value of only £5.73 when discounted at 10 per cent. The point is that the choice between the alternatives is being made at this point in time and *viewed from the present day*; outlays so far in the future will be insignificant if a positive rate of time preference is assumed. Those who desire more discussion of this point should consult Appendix 4.

be required. A similar situation occurs where the resource usage associated with two alternatives does spread over a number of years but is the same in each and every year, including identical capital outlays at the beginning of the projects. Here the results can be expressed on an annual basis, again avoiding the need to discount. However, for many comparisons of alternative treatments, discounting is likely to be required.

5.2. Allowance for the risk and uncertainty in costs and benefits

5.2.1. What are risk and uncertainty?

Both of these are related to our lack of a guarantee that events will go according to plan. That is, all costs and benefits occurring in the future can be viewed as *expected* rather than certain. Obviously, attempts to allow for this fact can improve the quality of information provided by the analysis.

The distinction between risk and uncertainty is not clear-cut but the term *risk* is usually used to describe a situation where, in deciding upon the chances of a particular event arising, one has a history of occurrence of that event. This can be consulted in forming one's view. For instance, one can form a view, based on past evidence, on the likely success of a given category of surgery.

The term *uncertainty* is usually used to describe the situation where one has little useful evidence upon which to form a view. For instance, what are the chances of discovering a cure† for cancer within the next five years? Here there is a history of failure in the search for a complete cure, but few would suggest that this history implies that no cure will ever be found, nor even that it will not be found soon.

Since risk and uncertainty have the same implications for evaluative procedures, they are dealt with together below.

5.2.2. Coping with risk and uncertainty

The method of coping with risk and uncertainty depends partly on its source. That uncertainty arising from the underlying medical technology is usually dealt with by engaging in empirical study. In this way the probability distribution of the main medical variables

---

† Here the term 'cure' is used in its absolute sense. No one would deny that degrees of 'cure' or alleviation of the condition have already been realized.

can be ascertained: e.g. survival times, complication rates, time to return to work, and so on. The information gleaned from empirical study may be summarized to arrive at mean values and variances for each of the main variables.

Of course the economic estimates are also subject to uncertainty. In respect of the resources used in health treatments, one normally thinks of inflation as an uncertain element likely to bring about a revision of plans in the future. In fact *general* inflation should not affect the choice between alternatives;† if alternative A is more cost effective than alternative B, and the costs of both rise by 20 per cent, then A would still be preferred on economic grounds. However, if either of two alternatives were more affected by

---

† At first sight, this does appear always to be the case. For instance, if the budget does not keep pace with inflation we may no longer be able to 'afford' our first choice of alternative or alternatives.

Suppose the choice were between the following four alternatives, all of which can be undertaken only in total (i.e. they are indivisible).

	Costs (£)	Benefits (£)	Benefits − costs (£)
A	80	130	50
B	80	140	60
C	50	90	40
D	150	230	80

Given a budget of £200 we would select alternatives C and D, giving a net benefit of £120.

However, after 20 per cent general inflation we have

	Costs (£)	Benefits (£)	Benefits − costs (£)
A	96	156	60
B	96	168	72
C	60	108	48
D	180	276	96

If the budget remains at £200 we would now select alternatives A and B (a net benefit of £132), since we can no longer 'afford' C and D. Of course the point is that the budget has been reduced *in real terms*, since it has not been increased to keep pace with inflation. In fact this is not a case of 'general' inflation at all, since the budget has not risen at the same rate as other prices. Note that we would find a similar result if, with no inflation, our original budget of £200 had been reduced by 20 per cent to £160.

inflation than the other, then our preference for one over the other might be reversed. These changes in *relative* price levels might be brought about by one of a number of factors, such as changes in tastes, technological change or depletion in the stocks of raw materials such as fossil fuels. Similarly, one might find that (on the benefit side) valuations of improvements in health may change over time, as the society becomes richer or as individuals' views on what is worthwhile in life change.

Clearly the possibility of such changes may be less amenable to empirical study. Depending upon the amount of information (past and present) concerning the variable in question, one can attempt to estimate a single *'expected value'*.

Thus, if next year's benefits from a particular treatment are considered to have a 30 per cent chance of being £140, a 40 per cent chance of being £160, and a 30 per cent chance of being £180, then,

$$\text{Expected value of benefits (£)} = 140(0.3) + 160(0.4) + 180(0.3)$$
$$= 160.$$

Of course, these estimates may be no more than guesses on the part of those undertaking the analysis and it may not be wise to generate single expected values in this way. An alternative ploy is to carry out a *sensitivity analysis*. That is, to provide a range of estimates based on differing assumptions about the values that particular variables are likely to take, without any attempt to condense them into a single 'expected' outcome. Buxton and West (1975) adopted this approach in their appraisal of alternative treatments for chronic renal failure. They considered that the values assumed by five key medical and economic variables were likely to affect the outcome of the appraisal. For each of the five variables, three estimates were given—a 'best estimate', indicating the most likely value, and 'high' and 'low' estimates, indicating the likely upper and lower bounds. The estimates were as follows:

1. Survival rate of patients.

	Hospital dialysis		Home dialysis	
	Up to 6 years (per cent)	Over 6 years (per cent)	Up to 6 years (per cent)	Over 6 years (per cent)
Best estimate	50	Survival rate, s, from 0–6 years extrapolated as $s = 1 - e^{-kt}$	63.4	Survival rate, s, from 0–6 years extrapolated as $s = 1 - e^{-kt}$
Low estimate	50	0	63.4	0
High estimate	50	As a normal cohort	63.4	As a normal cohort

2. Rehabilitation rate of patients (return to work by the date given).

	Hospital dialysis (per cent)			Home dialysis (per cent)		
	1 year	2 years	3 + years	1 year	2 years	3 + years
Best estimate	30	52	60	45	65	75
Low estimate	20	25	35	25	35	45
High estimate	50	60	77	50	70	90

3. Treatment costs (1972 prices).

	Hospital dialysis	Home dialysis
Best estimate	£5600 annually including capital costs	£1300 initially plus £3390 per annum
Low estimate	Half best estimate	Half best estimate
High estimate	Twice best estimate	Twice best estimate

4. *Average earnings of patients†* (*1972*).

Best estimate	£1908 per annum (males)
	£1066 per annum (females)
Low estimate	Half best estimate
High estimate	Twice best estimate

5. *Discount rate* (*per cent*).

Best estimate	10
Low estimate	6
High estimate	14

Buxton and West then calculated the cost–benefit ratios for home and hospital dialysis, using the differing estimates. The results are shown in Table 5.2; x indicates that the best estimate was used.

It can be seen that the 'best estimate' assumptions give cost–benefit ratios of 6.4:1 for hospital dialysis and 3.2:1 for home dialysis (top row of Table 5.2). However, depending on the

TABLE 5.2. *Results of a sensitivity analysis—chronic renal failure*

					Cost–benefit ratios	
Survival rate	Rate of discount	Treatment costs	Rehabilitation rate	Average earnings of patients	Hospital dialysis	Home dialysis
x	x	x	x	x	6.4:1	3.2:1
Low	x	x	x	x	7.4:1	4.0:1
High	x	x	x	x	5.8:1	3.0:1
x	High	x	x	x	7.0:1	3.5:1
x	Low	x	x	x	5.8:1	2.8:1
x	x	High	x	x	12.7:1	6.3:1
x	x	Low	x	x	3.2:1	1.6:1
x	x	x	Low	x	11.0:1	7.4:1
x	x	x	High	x	4.9:1	2.7:1
x	x	x	x	Low	12.7:1	6.3:1
x	x	x	x	High	3.2:1	1.6:1
High	Low	Low	High	High	1:1	1:1.8

Source: Buxton and West (1975).

† Earnings were taken as a measure of the benefit to society of the treatment (see the earlier discussion of this point in §4.1).

assumptions made concerning the values of the 5 key variables, the cost–benefit ratios for hospital dialysis and home dialysis vary considerably. Only given the most favourable assumptions is the community seen to 'break-even' or 'profit' from dialysis (cost–benefit ratios of 1:1 for hospital dialysis and 1:1.8 for home dialysis). Of course the definition of 'benefit' used here is very narrow. The most important category of economic benefit excluded is the value *per se* of the extension of life gained by dialysis. Buxton and West do not attempt to estimate this benefit directly. However, it is shown elsewhere in their paper that (given 'best-estimate' assumptions) the community must value this extension at £4720 per annum or more, as it provides these treatments. This value is estimated from the excess of costs over benefits for hospital dialysis, the more costly of the two alternatives.

5.2.3. Two pitfalls

First, in the appraisal of new treatments, there is often a tendency to form an 'idealized' view of the innovation. It is worth remembering that a procedure not operating *in situ* can give rise to many unforeseen problems. Problems of a technical nature can be minimized by thorough 'field testing' of the new treatment, but organizational problems are harder to predict and are unlikely to become evident until the new procedure is in operation.

Second, the procedure of allowing for risk and uncertainty by changing the discount rate is hardly a pitfall, but a practice to guard against. The practice is based on the argument that since higher returns are sought by private investors when higher degrees of risk are involved, a 'risk premium' should be added to the discount rate for more risky alternatives. Although the method has the advantage that it is relatively easy to apply it should be avoided because:

1. It confuses issues of uncertainty with those of time preference. (It is a useful mental exercise for the analyst to consider these questions separately).
2. Any adjustment to the discount rate affects all costs and benefits equally, whereas in practice the degree of uncertainty surrounding these may differ from one cost or benefit to another.

Major points from this chapter

1. The differential timing of the effects of health treatments needs to be taken into account in any appraisal.

2. The procedure of *discounting* to present values is recognized as the best way of doing this.

3. Costs and benefits occurring in the future should always be regarded as expected rather than certain.

4. Careful field testing of the alternatives can increase one's knowledge of some of the key variables in the appraisal. However, in some cases it will be necessary to explore how sensitive the final result is to changes in the values of the key variables.

REFERENCES

Buxton, M. J. and West, R. R. (1975). Cost–benefit analysis of long term haemodialysis for chronic renal failure. *Brit. med. J.*, **ii**, 376–9.
Cohn, E. J. (1972). Assessment of malaria eradication: costs and benefits. *Amer. J. tropical Med. Hyg.*, **21** (5), 663–7.

6

Decision rules and decisions

Once the economic appraisal has been completed, how does one compare alternatives on the grounds of economic efficiency? Consideration of this question has led to the formulation of a number of 'decision rules' which have gained fairly common use in cost–benefit studies in health care. Typically the analyst will calculate an index, such as the ratio of costs to benefits, for each of the alternative courses of action being appraised. The alternatives will then be ranked in accordance with the index. This chapter has been entitled 'Decision rules *and decisions*', since discussion of decision rules inevitably raises the question of the relationship of economic appraisal to the decision-making process. Following the scheme set out in Fig. 1.1 (Chapter 1), it is unlikely that the economic appraisal will be the only input to the decision-making process and therefore the use of a 'decision rule' in the appraisal will not normally imply that a particular decision should be made. This would only be the case if economic efficiency were the only criterion for choice between alternative courses of action. This point can be illustrated by reference to a recent study.

In their cost–benefit study of screening for spina bifida cystica, Hagard, Carter, and Milne (1976) calculated a 'benefit–cost index (BCI)', which was derived 'by dividing the total economic benefits which the screening programme would produce, by its total costs'.

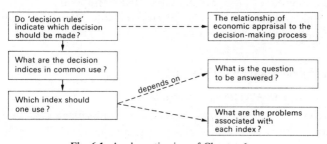

Fig. 6.1. A schematic view of Chapter 6.

Discounting future benefits and costs by 10 per cent, it was found that, owing to regional variations in the incidence of spina bifida births/1000 population, the BCI was less than unity for some areas. (In Birmingham (England), assuming incidence of 2.0/1000 total births and a screening test sensitivity of 40 per cent, the BCI is about 0.7.) Since the associated decision rule suggests that one should proceed only when the BCI is greater than unity, a naïve interpretation of this result would be that screening should not be instituted in Birmingham.

Fortunately, Hagard *et al.* (1976, p. 52) warn against this:

Such an eventuality might, but should not, be interpreted as implying that no case would exist for introducing screening in Birmingham . . . It is not a legitimate objective in this kind of exercise to maximise the BCI unless in association with the same or greater community benefits.

It appears that the point being made is that there are other benefits from screening, not incorporated in the index (i.e. the index is wrongly specified). Bearing in mind the difficulties in expressing all the effects of health treatments in commensurate units, this is likely to be a common failing of cost–benefit studies. This calls into question the wisdom of quoting indices as some people may accept them as an invitation to read no further.

In my view it is better to regard the calculation of decision indices merely as a convenient way of summarizing the information gleaned from an economic appraisal. Therefore, the use of decision indices should rest upon whether the analyst and the decision-maker feel that the economic information is best summarized in this way. The example cited above highlights the potential dangers in presenting a summary of only part of the relevant economic information. There are a number of other pitfalls associated with the use of some of the decision indices and these are discussed below, after a description of the indices in common use.

6.1. Some common decision indices

6.1.1. *In cost effectiveness analysis*

The cost effectiveness index expresses the results in terms of the cost to obtain a unit of the desired benefit, e.g. cost per year of life gained. An alternative with a lower cost effectiveness index (CEI) is preferred.

6.1.2. In cost–benefit analysis

Benefit–cost ratio (or index) (BCR) comes in two forms:

the *gross* $BCR = \dfrac{\Sigma \text{ benefits}}{\Sigma \text{ costs}};$

the *net* $BCR = \dfrac{\Sigma (\text{benefits} - \text{costs})}{\Sigma \text{ costs}}.$

Costs and benefits are discounted to present values where this is relevant. The two ratios are equivalent as the net BCR = gross BCR − 1. An alternative with a higher BCR is preferred. (Note that the ratio is sensitive to how one classifies the changes brought about by an alternative into 'costs' and 'benefits'. This problem is discussed later.)

Net benefit (or net present value) (NPV)

Net benefit $= \Sigma$ (benefits − costs)

Costs and benefits are discounted to present values where this is relevant. This index is known as *net present value* when the benefits and costs are discounted. An alternative with a higher (non-negative) net benefit (or net present value) is preferred.

Internal rate of return (IRR) derives directly from the formula for discounting costs and benefits:

Net present value $= \displaystyle\sum_{i=0}^{n} \dfrac{(B_i - C_i)}{(1 + r)^n}$

where r = discount rate, B_i = benefits in year i, C_i = costs in year i, and n = number of years. The internal rate of return is that value of r for which NPV = 0. The higher the internal rate of return of an alternative, the more likely it is to be preferred.

6.2. Which index should one use?

In choosing between decision indices it is important to note that there are three possible questions to be answered. These are:

1. Would undertaking the project be better than doing nothing?

2. Which of two mutually exclusive† projects (*X* and *Y*) should be undertaken?

3. How should projects *X*, *Y*, and *Z* be ranked when contemplating the prospect of an over-all budget constraint.‡

How do the various decision criteria fare in answering these questions?

6.2.1. *Would undertaking the project be better than doing nothing?*

Only the cost–benefit criteria are relevant here, since cost effectiveness studies do not attempt to provide an answer to this question. All three cost–benefit criteria appear to give unambiguous answers. Thus, undertake project *X* if:

    gross BCR(X) > 1;
    or net   BCR(X) > 0;
    or NPV (X) > 0;
    or IRR   (X) > the assumed rate of time preference.

However, there is a slight possibility of ambiguity with the IRR rule, as there is sometimes more than one solution to the expression for IRR.§

6.2.2. *Which of two mutually exclusive projects (X and Y) should be undertaken?*

All criteria give an answer here. Thus, undertake *X* not *Y* if:

    CEI(X) < CEI(Y)
    or BCR(X) > BCR(Y)
    or NPV(X) > NPV(Y)
    or IRR(X) > IRR(Y)

Here the use of the CEI and NPV criteria is unambiguous. However, there are potential problems with BCR and IRR. The main problem

---

† 'Mutually exclusive' means that if one of the two options is selected, then the other is automatically precluded.

‡ The constraint does not have to be a budgetary one; this is merely the most common manifestation of a resource constraint.

§ The calculation of IRR involves the solution of a polynomial equation. If the polynomial is of degree n, there will be n solution values of IRR, given by the roots of the equation. Although not all these will be real and positive (hence, providing admissible values for IRR) there will often be more than one such root, usually where costs exceed benefits in more than one year of the project.

with BCR is that the value of the ratio is sensitive to the designation of 'costs' and 'benefits'. Consider the following example.

A preventive programme requiring an outlay of £100 brings about savings in lost production of £120 and savings in future medical costs of £50. (Assume that these are all in present value terms—see Chapter 5.) One presentation of this result would be as follows:

$$\text{Costs} = £100$$
$$\text{Benefits} = £120 + £50$$
$$(\text{Gross}) \text{ benefit–cost ratio} = \frac{£170}{£100} = 1.7.$$

However, if the medical cost savings are treated as 'cost offsets' the result could be presented thus:

$$\text{Costs} = £100 - £50$$
$$\text{Benefits} = £120$$
$$(\text{Gross}) \text{ benefit–cost ratio} = \frac{£120}{£50} = 2.4.$$

The calculation of net present value has the advantage of giving the same answer in both cases:

Net present value $= £\{(120 + 50) - 100\} = £70$

or

Net present value $= £\{120 - (100 - 50)\} = £70$.

With IRR there is again the problem of multiple roots. A further complication arises where two mutually exclusive projects X and Y differ markedly in the *scale* of their initial capital outlay. Here, the IRR and NPV criteria can suggest different choices. Consider the following example.†

The excess of benefits over costs for two projects A and B is:

	Year 0 (£)	Year 1 (£)	Year 2 (£)
A	− 400	300	216
B	− 100	50	104

† Taken from Samuels and Wilkes (1971).

A has an IRR of 20 per cent and B has an IRR of 30 per cent. Thus a naïve interpretation of the IRR decision rule would suggest that B be preferred to A. Nevertheless, discounting at 10 per cent, A has an NPV of £51.2 and B an NPV of £31.4. Thus, by the NPV decision rule, A is to be preferred to B. What has gone wrong?

Since the two projects under consideration are mutually exclusive, the relevant question is whether it is worth making the incremental outlay of £300 in year 0 in order to receive higher benefits in the following two years. The conflict between IRR and NPV can be resolved by defining the *incremental project*, (A − B) the excess of benefits over costs for which are:

	Year 0 (£)	Year 1 (£)	Year 2 (£)
(A − B)	− 300	250	112

This has an IRR of 15.6 per cent. As this is greater than our rate of time preference, the rationale is that the extra £300 needed for A is well spent. Therefore, the NPV did give the 'right' answer in the first instance.

Thus, the arguments presented here suggest that one should follow the NPV rule when ranking two mutually exclusive projects.

6.2.3. How should the projects X, Y, and Z be ranked when contemplating the prospect of an over-all budget constraint?

Here the position can become quite complicated and it is unwise to use any of the simple rules. For instance these may give different rankings between a number of projects depending upon whether or not the projects are *divisible* (i.e. Does one have to undertake the whole project or can fractions of it be undertaken?) (The reader may remember that the indivisibility assumption was made in Chapter 5 in the footnote to §5.2.2. In the example given, would the position change if the indivisibility assumption were dropped? If so, why?)

The only universal approach to ranking under a constraint is through the use of *mathematical programming techniques*. These are outside the scope of this guide and the reader is advised to consult an expert.

Major points from this chapter

1. The 'decision rules' employed in economic appraisals

should not be interpreted as hard and fast rules for choice between health care alternatives.

2. The calculation of decision indices should be seen merely as a way of summarizing the results of an economic appraisal.

3. There are dangers in calculating a decision index when this does not encompass all the relevant economic information.

4. Net present value (or net benefit) is the most problem-free decision index. This should be used whenever a simple summary statement is required.

REFERENCES

Hagard, S., Carter, F., and Milne, R. G. (1976). Screening for spina bifida cystica: a cost–benefit analysis. *Brit. J. prevent. soc. Med.*, **38**, 40–53.
Samuels, J. M. and Wilkes, F. M. (1971). *Management of company finance*. Nelson, London.

7

Some case studies

In this chapter the principles outlined above are discussed in the context of four case studies. The four medical problem areas chosen differ considerably. These are: elective surgery, chronic renal failure, screening (with special reference to cancer control), and care of the elderly. In each case the purpose is not to discuss at length the actual results produced by studies, but to consider the ways in which the methodology of the existing work could be refined. Refinements are discussed under the following headings: improvements in the over-all design of the study, improvements in medical evaluation, improvements in cost estimation, and improvements in benefit estimation.

This discussion of refinements should not be taken as a plea for refinements *per se* on my part. It is important to question the purpose of refinements since they are likely to involve considerable time and effort. One should not necessarily aim to produce the best possible information every time. (To argue for this would be to suggest that economists commit the very sin that they attribute to others, viz. failure to count costs!) However, it is useful to identify possible refinements that ought at least to be considered, particularly in situations where such refinements:

(a) would broaden the scope of the study (say, to include extra alternatives, or to enable a 'higher level' question to be tackled); or
(b) might lead to different conclusions being drawn from the analysis (say, through the inclusion of better, or additional, information).

The over-all aim of this chapter is to give some indication of the different levels of complexity in economic analysis (and hence the different levels of confidence to be attached to study findings) even though for some purposes it may turn out that highly sophisticated analysis is not really required.

7.1. Elective surgery

Over the years there have been a number of changes in the pattern of surgical treatment. Along with the use of more highly technological medicine (a trend in common with other branches of clinical practice), there has been a trend towards shorter in-patient stays, and increasing use of day-case surgery or out-patient treatment for some conditions previously managed through a traditional in-patient admission. This change is probably the result of a wide variety of factors. Some of these relate to the benefits derived from care—patients may prefer to go home as early as possible, or the risks of cross-infection may be higher in hospital. Other reasons for change relate to resource use—individual clinicians may have modified their admission and discharge policies in response to pressures on beds or lengthening waiting lists. Whatever the reasons for change, the main question for economic analysis is whether or not these changes represent increases in efficiency. This question has been tackled by a number of analysts. Their work is discussed below and indications are given of the differing levels of sophistication in approach.

Using the terminology of Chapter 3, the study question being tackled is 'What is the most efficient way to treat a given condition?'. It will be remembered that under certain circumstances this question can be answered by employing the simpler form of the cost–benefit approach—cost effectiveness analysis. Taking the comparison of the effectiveness of treatment alternatives first, it could be argued that in the individual clinical context, slight adjustments in practice may be made over a period of time and the condition of patients carefully monitored so that one has data 'before and after' a change in policy. However, more rigorous assessment of the changes can only be obtained through carrying out controlled clinical trials. Consider, for example, the controlled trial carried out by Morris, Ward, and Handyside (1968), which compared periods of one day and six days hospital stay after the repair of inguinal hernia. It was found that 'although short-stay patients required some additional domiciliary care, the post-operative progress of patients in both groups was the same in other respects' (see Table 7.1).

Morris *et al.* note that 'the "acid test" of the efficacy of hernia repair lies in the development of recurrences'. At the time of reporting, 138 patients had been reviewed by the consultant staff, all at least twelve months after operation. Of these, 70 were in the

TABLE 7.1 (a) *Intercurrent illnesses developed by patients after operation*

Nature of illness	Short stay (92 patients)	Long stay (93 patients)
Chest infection	9	7
Wound infection	3	1
Haematoma (wound, scrotum, or spermatic cord)	3	5
Unexplained pyrexia	4	2
Thrombophlebitis	1	0
Dermatitis (reaction to dressings)	1	1
Pain at operation site	1	0
Others (back bain, faecal impaction, attack of asthma, laryngotracheitis, subconjunctival haemorrhage)	3	2
All illnesses	25	18

(b) *Intervals after operation at which intercurrent illnesses were diagnosed*

Nature of illness	Allocated stay	Time of diagnosis (post-operative days)			
		1	2	3	>4
Chest infections	Short	3	2	1	3
	Long	3	2	1	1
	Total	*6*	*4*	*2*	*4*
All wound complications	Short	3	1	0	3
	Long	4	1	0	1
	Total	*7*	*2*	*0*	*4*
All other illness	Short	5	1	1	2
	Long	3	0	0	2
	Total	*8*	*1*	*1*	*4*
All illnesses	Short	11	4	2	8
	Long	10	3	1	4
	Total	*21*	*7*	*3*	*12*

After Morris *et al.* (1968).

short-stay group and 68 in the long stay group. Recurrences were discovered in six patients, two in the short-stay group and four in the long-stay group. The authors conclude that 'the results of case review provide no evidence to suggest that early discharge is in any way more conducive to the development of recurrences than conventional periods of hospital stay'.

7.1.1. Improvements in medical evaluation

A controlled trial is the best kind of medical evidence upon which to base economic analysis, so the comments here will be brief. The most common criticisms of clinical trials are that the dimensions of effectiveness assessed are in some sense 'inappropriate', or that the follow-up period is not long enough, or that the method of allocation of patients to the treatment groups is unsatisfactory or that the numbers in the trial are too small. There is always scope for debate concerning these issues in respect of any trial—is long-term follow-up ever long enough? However, let us suppose that equivalence in medical effectiveness has been established in this case—a sufficient condition for simplification to the cost effectiveness approach. Given that the cost per in-patient week in acute hospitals (at 1978 prices) is around £200 per week, is it not obvious that treatment by the short-stay alternative must be more efficient? There are a number of possible refinements to this simple costing argument.

7.1.2. Improvements in cost estimation

Would a reduction of 5 days in the average length of in-patient stay of hernia patients save five-sevenths of £200? It would be unlikely to do so, for at least three reasons. First, average cost per in-patient week (as given in routine hospital cost statistics) is calculated from the expenditure generated by a heterogeneous mix of in-patient cases. Hernia cases may not be close to the 'average' case in terms of expense. Second, the majority of the costs of a particular acute surgical case will be generated in the first few days following admission, where the bulk of investigation and treatment takes place. The days of stay towards the end of a typical in-patient spell will be less resource intensive. The patient is likely to be consuming only 'hotel' services and basic nursing care (see Figure 7.1).

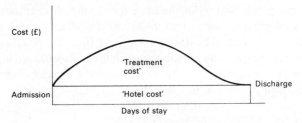

Fig. 7.1. The variation of hospital cost with hospital in-patient stay.

Finally, there is the *marginal* question. Precisely which costs would be escaped if stays for a few patients were shortened? Certainly not all the daily hotel costs, and possibly not all the treatment costs. For example, items such as general administration, medical records, and power, heat, light, are likely to be independent of patient stay. It is obvious that more sophisticated approaches are required in order to explore the resource consequences of a change in surgical policy.

Two methods are often used to combat the first two problems outlined above. The first is the statistical technique of *multiple regression analysis* which can be used to explore the systematic relationships between hospital cost per case (or per in-patient week) and various aspects of hospital operation, such as the types of cases treated, average length of in-patient stay, bed occupancy, and so on. Depending upon the variables fed into the model, average cost data can be obtained for broad specialty or disease groupings. In addition, 'hotel' costs can be separated out from 'treatment' costs.† The regression approach has been used with some success by DHSS to obtain estimates of average costs by specialty and an estimate of the saving from reducing length of stay. (This was found to be about £4.50 per day (1970 prices). Obviously this figure is much less than 1/7th of average cost per in-patient week. See Hurst (1977).)

---

† More precisely, the analysis separates those costs which are systematically related to length of stay from those which are not. The statistical analysis of hospital costs is outside the scope of this book. There are numerous pitfalls in the approach and the results of such analyses should be treated with some caution. For a discussion of some of the problems see Berki (1972) and for recent applications see Culyer, Wiseman, Drummond, and West (1978) and Hurst (1977).

An alternative approach is to attempt to cost particular types of cases by:

1. Identifying those hospital resources which are particular or *individual* to given patients and those which are *shared* with other patients.
2. Devising rules for apportioning shared costs between patients. (The most common method is to allocate shared costs in proportion to the number of days the patient stays in the hospital.)

Examples of this approach are the work by Babson (1973), in costing alternative treatments in maternity care and in costing appendectomies, Russell (1974) in costing the treatments of all the patients passing through a surgical unit during a six-month period, and Piachaud and Weddell (1972) in costing treatments for varicose veins.

The approaches—of regression and cost apportionment—can give more accurate estimates of the average costs of particular treatments. However, apart from the various methodological and practical problems that they present, neither of them tackles the third problem outlined above. That is, a change in surgical policy (such as shortening stays) may not enable one to escape all components of cost. In terms of the discussion given in §3.2, *marginal* costs (or in this case marginal savings) will differ from average costs. One approach to solving this problem has already been cited in §4.2.2. (Russell, Devlin, Fell, Glass, and Newell 1977). Here the savings from instigating day-case surgery for hernia and haemorrhoids were estimated on the basis that day-case surgery would either (i) enable a five-bed ward to be closed or (ii) enable construction of a new five-bed ward to be avoided. It was estimated that the saving from day-case surgery would be between £19 and £24 per case (1973 prices), depending upon which of these two outcomes resulted from the change in surgical policy.

An interesting extension of this approach is suggested by the work of Harper (1974). For example, it is quite likely that freeing beds for other uses (say, by shortening stays) will lead to an increase in patient throughput. Therefore, rather than the hospital experiencing cash savings from shorter stays, resource consumption may actually *increase* as a result of the change in surgical policy. The size of the (opportunity) costs resulting from the increased throughput will depend on the amount of spare capacity available in particular key 'resource areas', such as operating theatres, wards, and diagnostic departments. Thus, in the unlikely event that, say, radiographers were sitting around with no work to occupy their time, an increase in the throughput of patients would imply only that radiographers' leisure time is forgone! This is likely to represent a lower cost than if their services were denied to other patients as a result of the increased throughput. Of course, these opportunity costs of increased throughput will also appear as financial costs whenever extra capacity is 'bought in' to meet the increased demand. The fact that being more 'cost effective' (or efficient) may involve extra expenditure just reinforces the point that the efficiency, say, of shorter stays depends upon both costs and benefits.†

So far the argument concerning the efficiency of shorter stays has referred only to changes in *hospital* resource use. (Unfortunately, this is often the case.) Obviously, a more sophisticated approach to assessing the efficiency of the surgical alternatives would include consideration of those changes in resource use outside the hospital, e.g. in community services and patients' resources. This is particularly important if one has reason to believe that lower consumption of hospital resources is likely to be accompanied by higher consumption of these other categories of resource. Thus, day-case surgery may require patients to be visited by a community nurse on the evening of their discharge. Earlier discharge may also require an additional input of 'nursing' care in the home from one of the family. If that member of the family loses opportunities of work or leisure there will be an extra cost to be considered. In addition, the different surgical alternatives may bring about differences in the patient's ability to return to work although this is likely to be linked to medical effectiveness (which for the moment we have assumed to be equivalent).

Some of these additional changes may serve merely to reinforce the economic advantages of the least cost alternative. For example, in their study of alternative therapies for varicose veins, Piachaud and Weddell (1972) measured the patients' time taken up in treatment and the time taken for convalescence. These were,

† Harper's work is discussed in an annex to this section.

respectively, 30 hours and 6.4 days for injection-compression sclero-therapy, and 100 hours and 31.3 days for surgery. Since surgery had been found to be the more costly treatment, no attempt was made to place money values on these changes, as this was not necessary in order to decide upon the relative efficiency of the treatments.

So far surgical innovations have been discussed under the simplifying assumption that the alternative treatments are equally effective. How would one pursue the efficiency question if this assumption were relaxed? Of course it is a possibility that the least resource-intensive treatment is also the more effective, but how would one proceed if the reverse were true? There are two ways in which to grapple with this problem. One general route suggests improvements in the over-all study design, the other suggests improvements in benefit estimation.

7.1.3. *Improvements in the over-all study design*

One way to proceed would be to investigate whether the treatment population could be subdivided in some way so that, for particular *subsets* of patients, the two treatments would again be found to be equally effective. In the case of, say, varicose veins, the relative effectiveness of the two alternatives may depend on the severity of the condition. Therefore the question becomes one of identifying and measuring suitable *a priori* indicators of the effectiveness of treatment.†

However, even with disaggregation of the patient population, one may find that the more costly treatment is also the more effective for the majority of patients. This point is considered in the next section. However, it is sometimes possible to find an intermediate alternative, between the other two in terms of cost, but equally as effective as the more costly treatment. This was the procedure adopted by Russell *et al.* (1977), who, after finding that an 8-hour stay following haemorrhoid treatment by the Lord procedure produced twice as many complications, increased the length of stay to 24 hours (see Table 7.2).

---

† Incidentally, factors such as severity could also affect the relative costs of treatment. Therefore, if the patient population was divided into subgroups (say, by severity of condition) it would be necessary to re-examine the relative effectiveness and *costs* of alternatives by subgroup.

TABLE 7.2

	Planned length of stay		
	Day-case patients	Long-stay (trial patients)	Long-stay (excluded patients)
No. of patients	55	56	54
Complications (however slight)			
Hernia	12 out of 32	11 out of 35	17 out of 44
Haemorrhoids†	13 out of 23	6 out of 21	4 out of 11
Length of convalescence			
<4 wk	8	11	7
4–8 wk	22	21	12
>8 wk	14	12	12
Special arrangements made for			
return home	30	30	32
Average additional expenditure	£4.67	£5.12	£4.33
Preferred length of stay			
Shorter than occurred	2	11	1
Same as occurred	27	41	41
Longer than occurred	26‡	4	12
Average no. of GP consultations			
Home	0.87	0.55	0.60
Surgery	1.49	1.31	1.39
Average no. of DN visits	5.96	1.79	2.07

† Differences almost significant at 5 per cent level.
‡ Including 17 who would have preferred 24 hours.
Source: Russell *et al.* (1977).

7.1.4. *Improvements in benefit estimation*

If disaggregation of the patient population, or the search for an intermediate alternative, do not enable the simplifying assumption (of equal effectiveness) to be retained, one must face up to the question 'is the extra effectiveness worth the extra cost?' In Chapter 4 it was argued that one answer to this question lies in what the recipients of treatment would be willing to pay in order to receive the more effective treatment. In practice the answer to this question is likely to be hard to elicit, at least from the potential patients themselves who, if they are not actually going to be called upon to pay, would have an incentive to overstate their valuation of the extra effectiveness.

A slightly different approach would be to ask individuals to value, relative to one another, the 'health states' implied by the two levels of effectiveness. In the case of varicose veins the dimensions of health state might include factors such as levels of pain, mobility, and physical appearance. This approach is discussed in more detail in the next case study.

A completely different approach would be to compare the increases in effectiveness which would be achieved if a given amount of extra costs were incurred for therapy A, with what is being (or could be achieved) at the margin with the same resources when allotted to therapies B, C, or D. This would put decision-makers in the position of having an explicit framework for benefit evaluation, which in turn would enable a consistent pattern of decision-makers' valuations to emerge.

7.1.5. Concluding remarks

In the field of elective surgery it has been possible to base economic appraisals upon the results of controlled clinical trials. The major possibilities for refinements in approach are in the consideration of the costs of surgical alternatives and in the investigation of the precise resource changes resulting from changes in surgical policy. Because it has been possible to simplify the approach in situations where the alternative treatments are equally effective, analysis has often yielded unambiguous findings.

Annex to §7.1: Analysing the resource consequences of changes in surgical policy

An important first step in estimating the changes in resource use resulting from changes in treatment policy is the measurement of the amounts of key resources used by alternatives. The example given below is taken from the work of Harper (1974). Here the alternatives are treatments for five separate conditions, but equally these could be alternative treatments for the same condition. The resource units required for each alternative are given below, standardized for the number of patients (N) that could be treated in 100 bed days (see Table 7.3).

Table 7.3 can be interpreted as follows. If, through a change in surgical policy (or for any other reason), the number of admissions for (say) acute appendicitis were to fall by around 14 cases, 100 bed-days would be freed for other uses. What would be the conse-

TABLE 7.3 *Resource requirements of five surgical treatments*

Resource units required	Treatment				
	Acute appendicitis	Peptic ulcer	Varicose veins	Inguinal hernia	Carcinoma of the breast
Theatre (no. of minutes in theatre suite)	697	960	1717	1012	410
Drugs	3843	6231	2159	3747	2271
Wardcare (based on nursing dependency)	467	537	311	327	413
Radiography					
(a) minutes of radiographer's time	850	550	150	450	500
(b) no. of films	15	29	12	20	56
Chemical pathology	136	238	41	80	82
Haematology	102	130	98	84	166
Bacteriology	183	168	30	119	56
Pathology	136	84	—	25	118
Blood transfusion service (bottles of blood ordered)	136	973	—	100	649
Physiotherapy (units based on staff time)	48	53	9	56	40
ECG (no. of electrocardiographic strips)	—	2	6	8	3
Emergency surcharge (no. of out-of-hours calls)	17	12	—	4	4
Beds (no. of bed-days)	100	100	100	100	100
No. of patients (N)	13.6	8.9	31.9	21.1	5.7

quences of using these bed-days for other treatments? Approximately 9 peptic ulcer admissions would fill the beds but would have a differential impact on the use of other resources, e.g. more theatre time would be required, and so on.

The uses of this type of table are twofold. First, for surgical management purposes it can tell us where the pressures on resources are likely to fall owing to a change in policy (i.e. where are the major constraints?): it can also predict the likely impact of the policy change on the removal of cases from a given waiting list. Second, from the point of view of economic analysis, it is a step along the road to estimating costs and benefits. For example, if the change concerns the treatment of about 9 peptic ulcers at the expense of 13.6 acute appendectomies, the benefits of the change are those accruing from the treatment of the extra ulcer cases, plus those accruing from the resources freed in radiography (radiographer's time), pathology, bacteriology, and emergency cover.† The size of these benefits will depend upon the alternative uses to which the freed resources can be put. Likewise, the costs of the change are the 13.6 appendectomies foregone plus the costs resulting from the requirement for extra resources in theatre, drugs, ward case, X-ray films, chemical pathology, haematology, blood transfusion service, physiotherapy, and ECG. The size of these costs will depend upon whether these departments have spare capacity or whether resources will be diverted from other beneficial uses.

7.2. Chronic renal failure

Consideration of the economics of treatments for chronic renal failure is almost certain to arouse more emotions than the work in the field of elective surgery discussed above. Here one is quite clearly concerned with life and death and the problem area represents a more difficult challenge for economic analysis.

A useful starting point for this section is the study by Klarman *et al.* (1968), which has already been cited. This study set out to advise on 'the best mix of transplantation, home dialysis and centre (hospital) dialysis'. The comparison of *mixes* of treatment types is

---

† These are the resource areas where the requirement for 8.9 peptic ulcers is less than for 13.6 appendectomies.

the correct strategy since dialysis and transplantation are complements as well as alternatives. For example, patients often require dialysis while arrangements for transplantation are being made. In addition, if a transplanted kidney fails, patients may be returned to dialysis, permanently or temporarily, depending upon whether it is decided to attempt another transplant.

The study by Klarman *et al.* was of the cost effectiveness type, since it was not the intention to question whether treatment of this disease is worthwhile *per se*. It will be remembered from §3.1 that this restriction in scope means that the benefits of treatment need not be made commensurate with the costs. In this case the benefits of treatment were taken to be 'years of life gained', extension of life being taken to be the prime objective of treatment for this condition. It was found that the 3 basic treatment strategies differed in their cost per year of life gained (see Table 7.4).

TABLE 7.4

	Cost per year of life gained
Transplantation	$2,600
Centre dialysis	$11,600
Home dialysis	$4,200

Source: Klarman *et al.* (1968).

The lower figure for transplantation was primarily due to the longer survival time for patients with transplantation (17 years on average, compared with 9 years on average with dialysis). The difference between the two dialysis figures was due to the differences in the present value of the costs of maintaining patients on dialysis in the two locations. The authors conclude that 'transplantation is economically the most effective way to increase the life expectancy of persons with chronic kidney disease'. Given the evidence presented, this would appear to be a logical conclusion, and implies that, given a fixed budget, the number of years of life gained would be maximized by selection of the maximum transplantation route.

7.2.1. Improvements in the over-all design of the study

The over-all design of a study can be improved by recognizing the heterogeneity of the patient population. That is, although, say, transplantation is most cost effective over-all there may be subsets of the population for which it is *not* most cost effective, e.g. those patients whose lives may be put at serious risk by a surgical operation or those for whom a suitable kidney cannot easily be found (i.e. finding one would involve large costs in advertising, administration, tests, etc.). In principle one should be able to construct an *a priori* cost effectiveness index for each individual based on the likely costs and likely effectiveness of the various treatment methods. However, in practice one would find that patients could be grouped in accordance with bundles of particular characteristics—e.g. severity of condition, tissue type, age, and so on. Even then it may be that transplantation is found to be more cost effective than dialysis for all but a few subgroups.

The cost effectiveness position is much more likely to vary within the population with respect to the two dialysis alternatives. For example, some individuals may need more training than others in order to enable them to be dialysed at home. In addition, patients' home circumstances may vary. Both these factors, and possibly others, will give rise to variability in home dialysis costs. Although the present value of the cost of home dialysis may be lower than that for hospital dialysis, it is conceivable that for some categories of patient the position may be reversed. A more disaggregated study could investigate this possibility.

7.2.2. Improvements in the medical evaluation

Outcome data for chronic conditions usually has to be collected over a number of years. In the study cited, it was found necessary to collect survival data from a number of sources, to pool the data, and then to extrapolate. Nowadays there are longer-term data on survival under dialysis and transplantation, and these could be incorporated into a subsequent study.

In addition, there is no guarantee that the patients in the three groups are equivalent in all respects other than mode of treatment. In fact it is unlikely that they are. The best way of allowing for this would be to carry out a controlled clinical trial, allocating patients randomly to the treatment groups. Random allocation is ethically defensible when there is reasonable doubt as to the relative effectiveness of the various treatments. It may be, therefore, that in this case it would be unethical to allocate patients randomly between transplantation and dialysis (given the apparent superiority of transplantation), although it may be possible to allocate patients randomly between home and hospital dialysis.

The outcome measure is another major feature in the medical appraisal. Here the outcome measure is survival time, but there may be other factors to consider, such as the emotional strain of dialysis for some patients and their families, and the restriction of mobility that dialysis usually demands. Klarman *et al.* attempt to make allowance for differences in life-style between patients on dialysis and those with an effective transplanted kidney by valuing a year gained by transplant as equivalent to 1.25 years gained by dialysis.†

7.2.3. *Improvements in benefit estimation*

The attempt to adjust for the *quality* of the extra years of life gained (cited above) illustrates that the output from health treatments is hardly ever one-dimensional, i.e. measurement of the benefit in 'years of life gained' is not likely to give an adequate picture. There are two ways in which refinements in benefit measurement could proceed. First, an attempt could be made to value the health improvement in units commensurate with those used for valuing the resources (i.e. money terms). In this case the central question is one of valuing human life. The attraction of this approach would be that the scope of the study would be broadened to answer the question 'is treatment for chronic renal failure worthwhile *per se*?', or, in marginal terms, 'by how much should the dialysis and transplant programme be expanded?' One could proceed by considering values of life derived from other sources, e.g. the values people place on their own lives, derived from studies of what individuals are willing to pay for a reduction in the probability of their own death (e.g. Jones-Lee 1976), or the values awarded by courts to the relatives of deceased persons. (Of course, one problem here is that court awards represent an estimate of the value of a person's life not to himself but to others. The same could be said for the life insurance cover that individuals take out.) Alternatively one

† The researchers concerned would probably not wish to suggest that this adjustment is anything other than a crude method of allowing for the differences in 'transplanted' and 'dialysed' life-styles. However, since transplantation is found to be more cost effective in any case, the figure chosen does not influence the result of the study.

could merely present the decision-maker with the costs of expanding the programme set against the number of extra years of life gained. (See the comments on improvements in cost estimation given below.)

Second, instead of valuing the improvements in health in money terms, one could attempt to value one state of health *relative* to another. (This is the suggestion implicit in Klarman *et al.'s* assumption that one year gained by transplant is equivalent to 1.25 years gained by dialysis.) One method would be to approach the question directly, by asking questions like 'how many years on dialysis would you exchange for one by transplant?'. (This question could be asked of numerous groups in the community, not only patients and their doctors.) Alternatively, the question could be approached indirectly by identifying the key dimensions of health and asking individuals first to give *rankings of the* combinations of points on these dimensions (each combination being called a 'health state'), followed by relative valuations of the 'health states'.

An example of the latter approach from the work of Bush, Chen, and Patrick (1973) is given below (Table 7.5). Here particular health states are defined, each representing a particular combination of descriptive statements on 3 dimensions: mobility, physical activity, and social activity. Two groups of individuals were asked to assign weights to the different health states. These figures have been standardized using the end-points of 'death', value 0.000, and 'symptom-free', value 1.000. One can see that there is some disagreement between the consultants' and students' rankings. This highlights the point that individuals' values with respect to health vary. The variation between individual physicians is shown in another study (Torrance, Sackett, and Thomas 1973) (Table 7.6). Here, the health states to be valued relative to one another were identified as the actual regimens: home confinement, sanatorium confinement, kidney transplant, home dialysis, and hospital dialysis. The average values from the group of 11 physicians are shown in part (b) of Table 7.6. These indicate that for the group sampled, the utility of being given hospital dialysis is 58/83 (0.64) of being given a transplant. The equivalent figure for home dialysis is 56/83 (0.69).

The variations in the figures generated illustrate that such approaches are only at an experimental stage. However, in my view

TABLE 7.5 *Preference ratings (weights) for function levels, PKU consultants and graduate students*

Function level†	Mobility	Physical activity	Social activity	Preference rating	
				Consultants'	Students'
L30	Travelled freely (No symptom/problem complex)	Walked freely	Performed major and other activities	1.000	1.000
L29	Travelled freely (symptom/problem complex present)	Walked freely	Performed major and other activities	0.845	0.804
L28	Travelled freely	Walked freely	Performed major but limited in other activities	0.805	0.689
L26	Travelled freely	Walked freely	Performed self-care but not major activity	0.580	0.646
L24	Travelled with difficulty	Walked freely	Performed major activity with limitations	0.610	0.536
L17	Confined to house	Walked freely	Performed self-care but not major activity	0.435	0.594

L16	Confined to house	Walked freely	Required assistance with self-care	0.273	0.505
L11	Confined to house	In bed or chair	Performed self-care but not major activity	0.290	0.534
L10	Confined to house	In bed or chair	Required assistance with self-care	0.186	0.436
L9	In hospital	Walked freely	Performed self-care but not major activity	0.293	0.528
L8	In hospital	Walked freely	Required assistance with self-care	0.165	0.440
L7	In hospital	Walked with limitations	Performed self-care but not major activity	0.205	0.440
L3	In hospital	In bed or chair	Performed self-care but not major activity	0.152	0.428
L2	In hospital	In bed or chair	Required assistance with self-care	0.083	0.343
L0	Death	—		0.000	0.000

† Levels selected from classifications developed by Health Index Project.
Source: Bush *et al.* (1973).

TABLE 7.6
(a) *Utility values assigned to five health states by physicians using two methods. (Second values are results of replicated questions for each physician)*

Physician number	Home confinement		Sanatorium confinement		Kidney transplant		Home dialysis		Hospital dialysis	
	t†	p†	t†	p†	t†	p†	t†	p†	t†	p†
1	0.61	0.26	0.02	0.01	0.61	0.43	0.55	0.19	0.10	0.10
	0.47	0.11			0.82	0.43				
2	0.47	0.31	0.50	0.05	0.94	0.84	0.39	0.36	0.40	0.25
	0.52	0.31			0.82	0.79				
3	0.33	0.17	—	0	0.85	0.66	0.61	0.50	0.50	0.25
	0.50	0.33			0.78	0.68				
4	0.50	0.50	0.67	0.88	0.96	0.96	0.93	0.93	0.80	0.90
			0.75	0.88	0.98	0.98				
			0.75	0.42	0.78	0.85				
5	0.86	0.72			0.88	0.72	0.88	0.87	0.80	0.58
	0.79	0.86			0.88	0.50	0.92	0.87		
6	0.50	0.50	0	0	0.91	0.90	0.05	0.29	0.10	0
	0.50	0.42			0.94	0.90				
7	0.46	—	0.25	0	0.63	0.70	0.86	0.86	0.80	0.80
	0.56	0.70			0.74	0.70				
8	0.12	0.37	0.11	0.01			0.55	0.15	0.38	0.42
	0.37	0.25								

9	0.81	0.89	0.11	0.75	1.00	0.97	0.97	0.91	0.99	0.90
	0.91	0.96			0.97	0.99				
10	0.71	0.91	0.25	0	0.84	0.93	0.63	0.81	0.50	0.38
	0.85	0.91			0.92	0.97				
11	0.88	0.88	1.00	0.75	0.93	0.91	0.80	1.00	0.92	0.90
	0.90	0.88			0.92	0.91				

† t represents value measured by time trade-off technique; p represents value measured by von Neumann–Morgenstern standard gamble. (For more discussion see Appendix 3.)

(b) Average health state utility values

Health state	Utility
Healthy	1.00
Kidney transplant	0.83
Home dialysis	0.66
Home confinement	0.56
Hospital dialysis	0.53
Sanatorium confinement	0.34
Dead	0.00

Source: Torrance *et al.* (1973).

such work should be taken seriously if only for the fact that it exposes the value judgements implicit in assessing the relative contributions of therapies to health. To this end I discuss these approaches further in Appendix 3.

7.2.4. *Improvements in cost estimation*

In improving the cost estimates, it is important to ask whether any relevant costs have been omitted. In the study by Klarman *et al.* (1968), a particular concern is the underestimation of the costs of home dialysis. For example, resources may be required to adapt patients' homes for dialysis. In another study, Buxton and West (1975) found that the costs of adaptation varied considerably, but concluded that 'the most recent practice has been to install mobile caravan units at a cost of about £1300'. In addition they indicated that 'this figure has been used in the estimation of the cost of the home dialysis programme, since the 'cheaper' alterations were likely to be subsidized by patients' families by the provision of existing rooms for the equipment, and therefore they would probably have true costs as high as for the caravan units'. (For example, rooms are being denied alternative uses.) Another important omission in the study by Klarman *et al.* is the cost of domiciliary back-up for home dialysis. This may involve 'nursing' care provided from within the family. The size of this cost will depend upon the alternative uses of relatives' time.

Because of the links between the three major treatment alternatives, costing problems can become quite complex. For instance, transplantation will normally involve a certain amount of dialysis while patients are waiting for a kidney. Also home dialysis requires that a hospital dialysis centre be in existence as patients require to be trained in hospital before moving onto home dialysis. In addition, spare capacity needs to be built into the hospital facilities to accommodate home dialysis patients who may be re-admitted from time to time. Coupled with the fact that the costs of hospital dialysis may include an element of general hospital overheads, it is likely that the difference in cost between home and hospital dialysis is not as large as suggested.

Finally, if one were thinking of broadening the scope of the study to answer questions such as 'by how much should the kidney dialysis and transplantation programme be expanded?' a slightly different approach to costing would be required. This is because the marginal (or incremental) costs may differ from the average costs of the existing programme. For example, the study by Klarman *et al.* takes no note of the costs of obtaining kidneys. While it might be possible to obtain small numbers of kidneys fairly cheaply (although not at zero cost!), it is likely that the cost per kidney will increase as more kidneys are required, since greater amounts of resources would need to be devoted, say, to advertising and administration of a kidney donor scheme.

7.2.5. Concluding remarks

The discussion above indicates that many refinements could be made to the original study by Klarman *et al.* Some of the refinements identified may change the findings of the original study, others may confirm it. Furthermore, it is clear that local circumstances have a bearing on what is efficient—is there spare capacity in the hospital dialysis unit; what is the standard of housing locally and what would it cost to adapt patients' homes? Finally, it can be seen that broadening the scope of the study requires abandonment of the original cost effectiveness framework and that this introduces many extra complexities.

7.3. Screening (with special reference to cancer control)

Screening for disease is thought by many to be an attractive proposition and a logical extension of medical practice. Since many aspects of medical therapy are at present unsatisfactory, it would be valuable if earlier diagnosis made therapy more effective. Cochrane and Holland (1971), in a general discussion of the validation of screening procedures, acknowledge these attractions but add that there are at least three other points to be considered before initiating screening programmes. These are: (i) the ethical issues raised by screening; (ii) the quality of the scientific evidence about the effectiveness of the screening tests; and (iii) the financial consequences of screening.

The financial questions are taken as the starting point for this discussion of the economics of screening programmes. Cochrane and Holland calculated that in 1971 the cost of saving the life of a patient with porphyria variegata, by population screening, was around £250 000; yet community screening for the disease had never been tried in the USA or UK. They claim that this 'suggests a conscious or unconscious recognition of the financial factor'. In economic terms, since screening programmes divert resources from other beneficial uses, one must ascertain whether the benefits from screening exceed the costs. A number of attempts to answer this question have been made in the field of cancer control. This work is featured in the discussion below, but the lessons to be learned are equally applicable in other branches of medicine.

The simplest economic argument in favour of screening is based on the proposition that screening programmes will cut health service costs overall, since costly medical care for the more advanced stages of the disease will be avoided. This is the argument put forward by Schneider and Twiggs (1972) in a study of the costs of carcinoma of the cervix. Costs of cytology screening for carcinoma of the cervix are analysed and the expenses of medical care compared in three hypothetical populations: (a) unscreened; (b) screened for the first time; and (c) an ideal population screened repeatedly in the past. It is suggested that 'once all prevalent disease has been identified and treated, a reduced schedule in which patients are screened every third year is medically acceptable. Under these conditions, medical costs of carcinoma of the cervix become less than those in an unscreened population and there are no deaths from the disease' (see Table 7.7).

Therefore, can one conclude that screening for carcinoma of the cervix is worthwhile in economic terms? The epidemiologist would be likely to question some of the medical evidence upon which the study is based. Some argue that the link between carcinoma *in situ* (which is detected by the screening tests) and invasive cancer (which can result in death) is not adequately understood. In addition, it has not been possible so far to construct a satisfactory controlled trial of this screening procedure.

To these medical objections the economist could add a number of points concerning the economic methodology. In particular, no adjustment was made for the fact that, under the screening regimen, resources would be committed at an earlier stage. Following the arguments set out in Chapter 5, costs and benefits should be discounted to take account of their differential timing. The general effect of discounting by a positive discount rate would be to make most screening programmes less attractive from an economic point

TABLE 7.7

(*a*) *Annual costs of carcinoma of the cervix in a theoretical unscreened population of 100 000 women aged 20 or more*

	$
30 incident cases of invasive cancer of the cervix	
30 primary cancer therapy at $2800	84 000
15 further therapy and terminal care at $13,200	198 000
Total	282 000

(*b*) *Annual costs of carcinoma of the cervix in a theoretical population of 100 000 women aged 20 or more (screening every third year; patients previously screened regularly)*

	$
33 333 cytology smears at $5	166 665
66 cone biopsies for abnormal smears at $460	30 360
6 negative cones (excluded)	
60 carcinoma *in situ*	
39 treated by total hysterectomy at $1434	55 926
21 treated by wide conization at $460	9 660
Total	262 611

Source: Schneider and Twiggs (1972).

of view. Also, the economist would argue that some of the costs of screening have been omitted. For example, attendance for smears and for biopsies will involve patients in transport costs and will result in lost productive output or leisure time.

On the other hand, it could be argued that there are also time and production losses associated with the treatments for invasive cancer (which hopefully would be averted under the screening regimen). In addition it could be argued that women are reassured by being screened and that reassurance is of value.

Clearly there is considerable scope for more sophisticated approaches to examining the economic worth of screening programmes. These are examined below.

7.3.1. Improvements in over-all study design

There are a number of sophistications that can be built into a cost–benefit study of a screening programme. The first of these, mentioned above, is that the precise *timing* of costs and benefits should be identified so that discounting can be employed. It is often useful to set out this information in table form, as in the study of screening for spina bifida cystica by Hagard, Carter, and Milne (1976) (see Table 7.8). This is a shortened version of a table produced for an earlier paper (Hagard, Carter, and Milne 1975).

Here the costs of caring for 90 survivors with myelocele are set out for the present year (year 0) and for several years stretching into the future. (These costs would be averted if a screening programme were instituted and therefore form part of the benefit from screening for spina bifida cystica.) The effects of discounting by different rates can be seen. For example, the undiscounted cost of caring for the 47 children surviving until one year's time is £15 280 (second row of table, column (a)). Discounted (at 5, 10, or 15 per cent) this sum has a *present value* of £14 550, £13 890, or £13 290 respectively (row 2, columns (b), (c), and (d)). It can be seen that the costs in later years have very small present values when discounted, say, at 10 per cent. (In fact it could be argued that since these have little bearing on the result, the costs far into the future can be ignored altogether. For example, a cost of £26 200 occurring in 55 years time adds only £140 to the present value of costs if discounted at 10 per cent (last row of table, columns (a) and (c)).

Secondly, the over-all design of a screening cost–benefit study could be improved by considering a wider range of alternatives. One can consider 'population screening' and 'no screening' as end-points of the spectrum, and it is probable that while *population* screening may not be economic for some diseases, certain *selective* screening programmes will be. Some of the factors causing the cost–benefit position to vary between various subsets of the whole population will be medical—e.g. variation in the prevalence of the condition by age, sex, socio-economic group, or past medical history. Other factors may be non-medical. For example, it may cost more to screen some groups because extra resources need to be devoted (say, in education) to encourage them to participate in the screening programme. Whether or not such refinements are worth building into a study will depend upon how clear decision-makers are upon the policy options to be explored. For example, it may be the case that (on equity grounds) the screening programme is to be provided for all or for none. Alternatively, it may be that the most costly groups to screen are also the most underprivileged groups in

TABLE 7.8 Costs of caring for 90 survivors with myelocele

| | No. of survivors | | | Costs | | | | | | Additional costs | | | Present values discounted at | | |
| | Handicap category | | | Hospital treatment | | | | | | | | | | | |
Year	2	3–5	Total	In-patient	Out-patient	Physio-therapy	Permanent care	Education	Maternal income	Childhood	Adults	Total cost (a)	5 per cent (b)	10 per cent (c)	15 per cent (d)
				£	£	£	£	£	£	£	£	£	£	£	£
0	—	—	90	89 930	390	—	—	—	5 550	1 850	—	97 720	97 720	97 720	97 720
1	—	—	47	6 400	1 480	—	—	—	5 550	1 850	—	15 280	14 550	13 890	13 290
2	—	—	45	13 290	1 410	—	—	—	5 550	1 750	—	22 000	19 950	18 180	16 630
3	—	—	43	14 650	1 380	1 180	—	2 850	4 440	3 300	—	27 800	24 010	20 890	18 280
4	—	—	42	8 580	1 350	1 180	—	2 850	4 440	3 200	—	21 600	17 770	14 750	12 350
5	10	31	41	7 450	1 350	1 070	—	11 040	7 770	3 100	—	34 070	26 690	21 150	16 940
12	10	30	40	3 450	1 000	—	2 290	6 970	9 990	3 000	—	25 480	14 190	8 120	4 760
16	10	29	39	2 020	—	—	2 290	—	—	—	1 220	10 940	5 010	2 380	1 170
21	10	26	36	—	—	—	1 010	—	—	—	7 910	29 150	10 460	3 940	1 550
30	10	20	30	—	—	—	1 010	—	—	—	28 140	29 150	6 750	1 670	440
40	10	11	21	—	—	—	1 260	—	—	—	27 890	27 860	3 960	620	100
55	9	0	9	—	—	—	500	—	—	—	26 200	26 200	1 790	140	10
										Lifetime totals:		1 059 000	573 600	354 800	267 700

Source: Hagard, Carter, and Milne (1976)

the community. If health programmes are seen as a way of redistributing the nation's wealth in favour of these groups, then the extra weight given to benefits accruing to these groups may outweigh the extra costs (see Appendix 2). In any case, it is a legitimate role of analysis to ensure that such issues are approached systematically.

Thirdly, the study design has to recognize that the costs and benefits of screening programmes are related to the sensitivity and specificity of the screening test(s). In the cases of quantitative screening tests, there is latitude in the choice of the level at which the test is considered positive. If the level is chosen so that the test is highly specific (i.e. a high ability to give a negative finding when the individual does not have the disease or abnormality in question) the test is likely to have a lower sensitivity (i.e. the ability to give a positive finding when the individual screened does have the disease or abnormality under investigation). In short, aiming for fewer false positives is likely to lead to more false negatives, and *vice versa*. Most economic appraisals of screening programmes assume the level to be set exogenously, but it would be relevant to explore how the size and distribution of costs and benefits of screening vary with different levels. This is the economist's way of expressing Cochrane and Holland's (1971) point that . . .

the decision on the screening level used must ultimately rest on a subjective judgement of the number of false positives and false negatives which would be tolerable to the population and the providers of the screening service. This judgement should, however, be based on the severity of the disease, the cost of the test and the time taken to administer it, and the advantages and probability of early treatment.

The estimation of the pay-off in economic terms from improved screening tests—that is, tests that are, say, more sensitive without being less specific—would provide an additional bonus from this broad approach.

Exploration of the variation in costs and benefits with test and population characteristics is greatly helped by a more formal expression of the relationships between all these factors. A useful formulation of the breast cancer screening 'problem' in cost–benefit terms is given by Kodlin (1972).†

7.3.2. Improvements in medical evaluation

Screening programmes are notoriously difficult to evaluate medically, for both practical and ethical reasons. Any uncertainty surrounding the medical aspects of screening inevitably filters through to the economics. In the absence of satisfactory controlled trials, the main way forward is to perform a sensitivity analysis along the lines suggested in Chapter 5, and to recognize that the costs and benefits estimated are only as good as the medical 'guesses' upon which they are based. In the meantime, the identification of the costs of particular screening programmes serves as a rough-and-ready guide to the urgency of answering some of the medical questions surrounding them.

7.3.3. Improvements in cost estimation

There are two important improvements in cost estimation that can be built into the appraisal of screening procedures. Firstly, the costs

---

† For example, the total cost of the screening strategy is defined as:

$$C_1 = P\pi_1[t + w + s] + P(1 - \pi_1)[t^1 + w + s] +$$

$$\text{(True positive)} \qquad \text{(False negative)}$$

$$+ (1 - P)(1 - \pi_2)[w_0 + bw_1 + s] + (1 - P)\pi_2[s]$$

$$\text{(False positive)} \qquad \text{(True negative)}$$

where P is the presumed frequency of breast cancer in the population, π_1 is the conditional probability of identifying a case correctly by mammography and palpation alone, π_2 is the conditional probability of identifying a non-case correctly, t is the treatment cost for a true positive (say, simple mastectomy), t^1 is the treatment cost for a false negative (say, radical mastectomy and radiation treatment), w_0 is the physical examination cost, w_1 is the biopsy cost, $w = w_0 + w_1$, s is the screen test cost, and b is the biopsy rate amongst false positives.

Similarly, the cost of a 'conventional' strategy is defined as

$$C_2 = P[t^1 + w] + \Phi(1 - P)[w'']$$

(women presenting   (women with no symptoms
with symptoms)   presenting for a check-up)

where t^1, w, P are defined as before, Φ is the 'worried well': the fraction of the non-diseased presenting for a check-up, and w'' is the work-up cost of the 'worried well' cases.

which patients incur in attending screening sessions are frequently omitted from appraisals, but should ideally be included. These costs will be made up of a money element (e.g. transport costs) and a time element. If working time is lost, one would need to include (as a cost) any losses in productive output. However, if the screen only involves a short absence from work, these losses might be quite small. Loss of leisure time also represents a cost to the patient. Similar arguments apply to the benefits from screening—there may be patients' costs and production losses associated with therapy as the condition progresses to the symptomatic state, and these may be averted by screening. Time costs were taken into account in a cost effectiveness study of the Pap test for cervical cancer by Schweitzer (1974). He estimated that the Pap test requires $1\frac{1}{2}$ hours total patient time (including waiting time, travel time, and procedure time) and that the diagnostic biopsy takes 2 hours. Assuming that the tests are performed by themselves and not in conjunction with other services and taking $3 as the average hourly wage of women employed full-time,[†] the time costs associated with the Pap test and punch biopsy were $4.50 and $6.00 respectively (1970 prices). (These compared with laboratory costs of $12 and $36 respectively). Similarly, for the cone biopsy, which demands one day of hospitalization plus two days of incapacitation, a rate of $78 per hospital day was assumed, plus $24 per day time cost.

Secondly, the use of average cost (per test) of a given screening programme often gives a poor guide to the costs of more extensive programmes. One reason, that in some cases extra resources may be required to encourage higher levels of participation in the programme, has already been suggested. (This would imply increasing marginal cost with increased programme size.) Another reason, which implies decreasing marginal cost, is that screening programmes may have set up costs (in the form of laboratories, equipment, and mobile units) that would not increase with higher levels of utilization. Therefore one cannot always predict whether a more extensive programme will cost more or less per test on average and it may be necessary to consider specific proposals in detail.

---

† Schweitzer assumes that those women not in the labour force will still have to hire temporary help.

7.3.4. *Improvements in benefit estimation*

It will be remembered that the simplest financial argument in favour of screening programmes is that they cut health service expenditure overall. However, in practice this is often not the case. Even if the analysis were widened to include non-health service resource use, as indicated in §7.3.3 above, screening may still not appear to be worthwhile merely in resource terms. It is likely that in many cases one would need to estimate the real health benefits of screening before it could be shown to be worthwhile in economic terms.

Where suitable medical evaluation can be carried out it would be possible to measure some of the changes in health state brought about by screening. These can then be set against the net resource cost implied by screening. For example, in his cost–benefit appraisal of cytologic screening for cervical cancer at the Mayo Clinic, Dickinson (1972) estimated that between 1960 and 1967, 184 screened and treated patients 'lived (on average) an extra 3.23 years, and that each additional year of life costs about $291'. This information is clearly of use to those who must decide whether or not screening should be instituted. For instance, they could compare these figures with the implied cost of extending life in other health programmes. Or, using a value of life derived from another source, they could decide whether enough resources in total were being employed in these life-saving activities.† In the case of screening for cervical cancer, one could raise serious doubts about the quality of medical evidence, but the approach could be used where more reliable data on life extension is available; for example, in breast cancer screening (Venet, Strax, Venet, and Shapiro 1971; Shapiro *et al.* 1973).

Of course, the benefits from screening are not confined to those individuals whose lives are extended. In addition, benefits accrue to a much wider group of individuals (the true negatives) who gain reassurance from being declared symptom-free.‡ The fact that the individual incurs costs (in time and expense) in obtaining the screen indicates that he or she makes an *ex ante* assessment that the screen

---

† These arguments are discussed at length in Chapter 4.

‡ Of course, this benefit is partly offset by the costs, in terms of extra anxiety, resulting from false positives and false negatives.

is worthwhile.† Remember that in Chapter 4 it was stated that one way of estimating the value of a programme to individuals is to ascertain the amount that they *would be willing to pay*. In the case of screening, it is possible to obtain information on what individuals have actually paid (in terms of time, energy, and travelling expenses).‡ The amount paid will vary between individuals, depending upon the distance travelled and mode of travel. The fact that the group of individuals who travel further pay a higher price to be screened gives rise to one method of estimating the benefits from the programme. If one could assume that those screened represented one homogeneous group, then those living nearby, paying a lower price, have not been called upon to pay an amount equal to what they would have been willing to pay. Therefore they experience a net gain. Of course it may be that individuals living in areas of differing distance from the service also differ in other important respects, e.g. income, attitudes to screening, and access to alternative services. In such cases, a more complicated form of the analysis is required. The general approach to measuring benefits described above has been used extensively in the field of leisure and recreation and a good introduction is given in Williams and Anderson (1976, Chapter 9). Clearly it has possibilities in the field of screening.

7.3.5. Concluding remarks

Economic analysis in the field of screening has shown that, by and large, screening programmes are not likely to be justified merely by their impact on health service resource use. It is usually necessary to calculate a wider set of costs and benefits. This case study indicates that many studies ignore both the non-health service costs of screening and the differential timing of costs and benefits. In addition, there has been little investigation of the value of the reassurance that screening programmes give, and one method of tackling this question has been suggested. However, the major stumbling block to the usefulness of economic appraisal in this field

---

† A possible exception to this is in cases where the individual is instructed to obtain a screen (say) by his doctor or by his employer. In such cases it would be interesting to examine the degree of compliance with such instructions.

‡ Remember that family and friends may also obtain reassurance from an individual being screened. In principle it would be possible to examine their 'willingness to pay' too.

is the lack of suitable medical evaluation. Ideally, economic appraisal would be more closely linked to such evaluation in the future.

7.4. Care of the elderly

So far much of this chapter has been devoted to the treatment of acute conditions, where the objective of care has been the control or cure of a specific condition. However, an increasing amount of health care resources are now devoted to the care of chronically sick and disabled persons, many of whom are elderly, who suffer conditions which are usually irreversible. Nevertheless, these conditions are the subject of alternative treatment regimens which yield differential benefits, in terms of the alleviation of the problems that the condition presents. Since these alternative regimens also have differential costs, they provide scope for economic appraisal. In contrast to some of the previous examples, there have been few, if any, controlled clinical trials of these alternatives, probably because of the enormous problems encountered in the measurement of the 'success' of therapy. Nevertheless, care of the elderly is seen as an important area by economists since, with an ageing population in many developed countries, increasing amounts of scarce resources are likely to be employed in the care of this client group. In addition, the great degree of fragmentation in the responsibility for care, between the health service, local government, and the family, suggests that the economist's wide perspective might yield additional insights.†

A detailed study of the relative costs and benefits of domiciliary care and local authority residential care, carried out by Wager (1972) for Essex County Council provides a useful starting point for the discussion of policies for the care of the elderly. The study put forward the tentative finding that in general elderly people will experience more satisfaction if they are maintained independent in their own homes for as long as possible. This is in line with the general government policy on health care priorities for the elderly in England (DHSS 1976, 1977). However, Wager (1972, p. 63) pointed out that

† For example, fragmentation implies that there is scope for one party to shift costs onto the others, with the possibility of inefficiency arising.

no age group is homogeneous in its motivations, and a humane policy must cater for the minority. Thus, it has been found that ex-service personnel or domestic staff who have spent a lifetime in communal living may positively prefer this way of life in old age, irrespective of their capacity to remain independent. Also, the decision on the extent of domiciliary care provided must have regard to the consequent demand on resources and competing needs.

The relative costs of domiciliary care and residential home care were calculated to establish the cost differences, excluding the costs of the various domiciliary health and personal social services, in order to identify the scope for providing more intensive domiciliary care to those who would benefit from it. The general idea was that, assuming a broad preference for domiciliary care on benefit grounds, one could allow the cost of domiciliary care to rise to the level of that for residential home care without being inefficient. The two relevant sets of costs (1970 prices) are given in Tables 7.9 and 7.10.

TABLE 7.9 *Comparison of the costs of accommodation*

	Average resource costs† per person per week	
Type of accommodation	Using 10 per cent‡ discount rate (£)	Using 5 per cent discount rate (£)
Residential accommodation	17.00	14.00
Old people living in 'normal' housing on their own		
Higher value, e.g. detached 3 bedroom house	19.50	14.00
Medium value, e.g. semi-detached 3 bedroom house	15.50	11.00
Lower value, e.g. semi-detached 2 bedroom house	13.00	10.00
Old people living in 'normal' housing with others	5.50–7.00	5.00–6.00
Old people's flatlets with warden (single person) or attached to residential home	13.50–14.00	11.00–11.50

† Wager uses the term 'resource cost' in the same way as the term '(opportunity) cost' is used in this guide.

‡ The discount rate was used to impute a weekly accommodation charge, or rental, from the capital value or capital costs of the various types of accommodation (see Wager 1972 for more details).

TABLE 7.10 *Average costs for domiciliary services*

Home help	42.1 p per hour
Meals-on-wheels	12.5–23 p per meal
Home nursing	69 p per visit
Health visiting	61.3 p per visit

In addition, it was known from a survey of old people waiting for residential accommodation that the costs of domiciliary health and personal social services currently given to most of them (92 per cent) totalled less than £3 per week. As the difference in the average weekly resource costs between residential accommodation and domiciliary accommodation was greater than £3 for most groups, it was recognized that it would make sense *on economic grounds* to intensify domiciliary care in order to maintain a person's ability to remain in the community.† There are several ways in which this major study could be refined.

7.4.1. Improvements in over-all study design

Domiciliary and residential care are two broad alternative methods of caring for the dependent elderly. However, hospital care is another legitimate alternative for this care group and it would be quite easy in principle to widen the scope of Wager's study by the inclusion of this third alternative. In fact, when thinking of the care of the elderly population as a whole, it is best to consider alternative *mixes* of the three forms of care. This point will be returned to later.

In addition it should be noted that there are many different alternatives within each major form of care. These would be worthy of more detailed investigation—e.g. the alternative methods of using home helps, of providing meals to someone who cannot cook, or organizing residential and long-stay hospital care. Furthermore, there are additional alternatives involving the use of day hospitals or day centres. (However, the discussion here will concentrate on the choices between the major forms of care.)

Returning to the question of the mix between the three major forms of care, a further refinement in analysis would recognize that the costs of providing domiciliary support or residential care will

---

† Provided that the increased domiciliary care would make the elderly person at least indifferent between domiciliary and residential accommodation.

differ from one elderly person to another. The costs will depend upon many factors—Wager's (1972) study showed that the type of domiciliary accommodation affected costs.† Probably the most important influence on cost levels is likely to be the level of disability or dependence of the elderly person. One could imagine that on a rising scale of disability (or dependence), domiciliary care could be the cheapest at low levels, only to rise above the costs of the other forms of care as disability increases (see Fig. 7.2).

The actual shape of these curves is not crucial to this discussion—merely the suggestion that they cross. Thinking of the whole client group as consisting of a number of subsets, with differing levels of disability or dependence, it is likely that the least cost form of care will vary between subgroups.

An interesting development from the notion of the intersecting cost curves is that one could think of a similar set of curves reflecting the benefits from, or the effectiveness of, the different forms of care. That is, there would come a level of disability or dependence where it would be better for the patient and/or for the family‡ if the patient were transferred, say, from the domiciliary regimen to the residential home regimen. Mooney (1978) has studied such patients, *at the margin* between two forms of care. He found that health care professionals were able to identify patients at each of the margins. Mooney goes on to suggest that one should

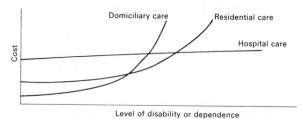

Fig. 7.2. Alternative forms of care for the elderly: the variation of cost with level of disability.

† Thus, the resource (or opportunity) cost implied by an elderly person occupying a large, high-valued house is higher than that implied by an elderly person occupying a room in a house shared with relatives.

‡ Of course, it is worth recognizing that what the family may prefer is often not what the patient may prefer. (This point relates to the distribution of costs and benefits—see Appendix 2.) Also see the discussion of family costs in §7.4.3.

concentrate the investigation on such marginal clients, in order to estimate the costs of caring for them in each form of care at the margin, and to ask decision-makers (the health care professionals in this case) to trade off the likely benefits of a move from one form of care to another against any increased cost. An important product of this approach is the identification of the bundles of characteristics pertaining to patients on each of the margins. For example, the kinds of characteristics identified are given in Table 7.11.

7.4.2. Improvements in benefit estimation

The identification of patient-related characteristics leads naturally to a discussion of possible refinements in benefit estimation in this

TABLE 7.11 *Health visitor community weighted population (7006 in toto)*

Characteristics	Percentage of population having listed characteristics		
	Not on 'margin' (N = 5685)	Residential home 'margin' (N = 1015)	Hospital 'margin' (N = 433)
Age†‡ 65–74	44.6	25.9	41.3
75–84	46.3	55.2	39.5
85 and over	9.1	19.0	19.1
Living alone†	41.8	74.6	40.3
Acute illness in last month‡	11.2	10.2	31.1
Incontinent‡	3.7	8.1	27.1
Instability (frequent falls)†	12.5	34.8	28.5
Night confusion†‡	2.3	19.9	54.3
Locomotor difficulties†‡	21.8	50.6	69.1
Mental impairment†‡	10.3	41.4	68.0
Self-neglect†‡	6.6	28.3	42.5
Tendency to isolation†‡	5.1	21.7	37.1
Unable alone with personal care†‡	20.0	45.2	83.7
Mobility unable alone			
out of bed†‡	14.4	25.4	60.3
in the house†‡	17.2	27.0	62.2
on stairs†‡	31.9	47.9	75.9
out of doors†‡	34.3	54.8	71.5

† Differences between RH margin and non-margin significant at 1 per cent level.
‡ Differences between hospital margin and non-margin significant at 1 per cent level.

Source: Mooney (1978).

field. Obviously, the relative benefits of different forms of care are crucial to the development of policies for the care of the elderly. Ideally one would like to: (a) specify the main dimensions of benefits; (b) measure the changes along these induced by particular forms of care; (c) devise a system of weighting the changes along each of the dimensions to arrive at an over-all index of the improvement in health state arising from particular regimens.

From a consideration of statements of objectives of social policy for the care of the elderly, Wright (1974) concluded that 'the major components that would need to be taken into account in a comprehensive measure of output would appear to be:

(a) Maintenance of independence;
(b) Maintenance or improvement of personal health;
(c) Social integration;
(d) Physical well-being or nurture;
(e) Compensation for disability.'

Unfortunately, progress so far has been slow, the major success being in the measurement of changes in health status and independence (Wright 1978). Moreover, the measurement of disability or dependency has not proceeded beyond ordinal measurement scales, either by using professional assessment or Guttman scaling (Williams, Johnston, Willis, and Bennett 1976). Thus multidimensional measures of benefit for programmes concerned with the care of the elderly are not yet at the same stage of development as those benefit measures discussed in the case study of chronic renal failure (Tables 7.5 and 7.6).

7.4.3. Improvements in cost estimation

If improvements in benefit estimation are developing slowly, what about the possible improvements in cost estimation? Better costing would still be of considerable use if one adopted the approach of subdividing the whole patient group into smaller groups, for which particular alternative forms of care were considered by professionals to be broadly equivalent, or if one supposed that two alternatives yielded differential benefits and that these needed to be set against costs.

The first set of refinements relate to the range of cost items typically considered. In the care of the elderly, a considerable burden can fall upon relatives and friends. Wager (1972) considered some of these costs, in imputing a rental for the room(s) occupied by elderly persons living with relatives. However, relatives and friends can provide considerable informal help and the problem is to decide whether or not it is given willingly. That is, time spent in helping an elderly friend or relative represents a cost (in that something, albeit leisure, has to be forgone†) but may also confer benefits on the helper. Probably all of us would be willing to devote *some* of our time to such a purpose; the question is whether helpers devote more time than they would ideally like. If this is the case, it is likely that devoting the time represents a net cost to them.‡ Therefore, this cost should, in principle, be taken into account.

Another element of resource use, often treated by the health sector as being 'free', is voluntary labour. This can be a key element in the care of elderly persons. The size of the cost involved depends upon the alternative uses to which this voluntary time could be put. Is an expansion in the use of voluntary labour denying the use of the same labour to other needy groups? If so, the cost is the value of the resources in their best alternative use. If volunteer helpers offer help for a specific purpose (e.g. to deliver meals-on-wheels) then the opportunity cost is small or even zero.

The second set of refinements relate to the *marginal* issues with which the reader should now be familiar. That is, the current *average* costs of caring for the elderly in each of the main regimens may not be relevant either to the switching of patients at the margin from one regimen to another, or to expansion of the different types of care. The kind of questions that one would need to ask are:

What will be the costs of (say) expanding hospital care and reducing residential care?

Will the resources freed in residential care be re-employed elsewhere—for example, in the care of the mentally handicapped—or are they specific to the care of the elderly and hence have a zero opportunity cost?

† Of course, it may be that work time is forgone. In the short run this will involve loss of earnings and/or productive output; in the long run it may involve loss of career opportunities.

‡ This is evidenced by the desire of some relatives to have an elderly person placed in an institution.

Given the increasing population 65 or over, what are the comparative costs of alternative expansion plans for both hospitals and residential homes?

Do increases in the scale of domiciliary services imply additional overhead expenses, such as those relating to administrative and supervisory staff, or office accommodation?

Obviously some of these questions could only be answered with any degree of precision when specific proposals are being considered. However, it is the notion of marginal costs being different from average costs that has overriding importance.

7.4.4. Concluding remarks

Progress in measuring the benefits resulting from alternative programmes for the elderly has been slow—mainly because of the multidimensional nature of the output and the lack of controlled clinical evaluations. However, a number of good quality costing studies have been carried out. These can be of use, first, because of the fragmentation of responsibility in the care of the elderly, and second, to enable alternatives to be compared on cost effectiveness grounds for carefully defined subsets of the whole elderly population.

7.5. Some lessons from the case studies

Although the case studies have been drawn from widely differing areas of clinical practice, several common points emerge.

1. In almost all cases there is scope for improvement in the estimation of the changes in resource use brought about by treatment alternatives. In particular:

(a) In rectifying omissions. (This applies especially to the resource consequences outside the hospital.);

(b) In recognizing the distinction between average and marginal costs or savings;

(c) In tackling the problems posed by the joint use of resources, especially in the hospital;

(d) In thinking of reductions in resource use not only as money sums to be saved, but as freed resources which could be redeployed.

In most cases, such refinements are not merely of methodological interest but are also likely to change the conclusions of the study concerned.

2. Given the relatively unambiguous nature of the results generated by studies of the cost effectiveness type, much could be gained from more extensive appraisal of alternatives that can be shown to be equivalent in terms of medical outcome.† This is a challenge for both economists and the relevant technical experts. While it is unlikely that many cases of precise equivalence of outcomes can be established for *the whole patient population* it is much more likely that cases can be found where this condition holds for particular *subsets* of that population.

3. In situations where the question being tackled has required the explicit valuation of changes in health state, the main contribution of economic appraisal to date has been in the calculation of the resource costs of obtaining such changes, so that these costs can be compared with those required to obtain similar changes in health state by alternative methods.

4. The value of economic appraisal is much reduced when there is a lack of reliable medical evidence. In such situations, its main role in the short term may be to obtain an accurate estimate of the costs of under-evaluated treatment programmes in order to highlight areas where the medical research effort should be intensified.

REFERENCES

Babson, J. H. (1973). *Disease costing*. Studies in Social Administration. Manchester University Press.

Berg, R. L. (Ed.) (1973). *Health status indexes*. Hospital Research and Educational Trust, Chicago.

Berki, S. E. (1972). *Hospital economics*. D. C. Heath and Co., Lexington, Kentucky.

Bush, J. W., Chen, M. M., and Patrick, D. L. (1973). Health status index in cost effectiveness: analysis of a P.K.U. program. In *Health status indexes* (ed. R. L. Berg). Hospital Research and Educational Trust, Chicago.

Buxton, M. J. and West, R. R. (1975). Cost benefit analysis of a long-term haemodialysis for chronic renal failure. *Brit. med. J.*, **ii**, 376–9.

Cochrane, A. L. and Holland, W. W. (1971). Validation of screening procedures. *Brit. med. Bull.*, **27** (1), 3–8.

Culyer, A. J., Wiseman, J., Drummond, M. F., and West, P. A. (1978). What accounts for the higher costs of teaching hospitals? *Social econom. Administration*, **12** (1), 20–30.

DHSS (Department of Health and Social Security) (1976). *Priorities for health*. DHSS.

† In fact all that needs to be shown is that the less costly alternative is *at least as effective* as the more costly alternative.

DHSS (Department of Health and Social Security) (1977). *The way ahead*. DHSS.

Dickinson, L. (1972). Evaluation of the effectiveness of cytologic screening for cervical cancer: III cost-benefit analysis. *Mayo Clin. Proc.*, **47**, 550–5.

Hagard, S., Carter, F., and Milne, R. G. (1975). *A cost-benefit analysis of screening for spina bifida cystica: methodology and detailed tabulations*. (Mimeo.) December.

——, ——, —— (1976). Screening for spina bifida cystica: a cost-benefit analysis. *Brit. J. prevent. soc. Med.*, **30** (1), 40–53.

Harper, D. R. (1975). *Comparative disease costing in surgical patients*. MD Thesis. Department of Community Medicine, University of Aberdeen. [Also summarized in Harper, D. R. (1979). Disease cost in a surgical ward. *Brit. med. J.*, **1**, 647–9.]

Hurst, J. W. (1977). Saving hospital expenditure by reducing in-patient stay. *Government studies in economics*. HMSO, London.

Jones-Lee, M. W. (1976) *The value of life: an economic analysis*. Martin Robertson, London.

Klarman, H. E., Francis, J. O'S., and Rosenthal, G. D. (1968). Cost effectiveness analysis applied to the treatment of chronic renal disease. *Med. Care*, **6**, 48–54.

Kodlin, D. (1972). A note on the cost-benefit problem in screening for breast cancer. *Methods Inform. Med.*, **2**, 242–7.

Mooney, G. H. (1978). Planning for balance of care of the elderly. *Scottish Journal of Political Economy* (June) **25** (2), 149–64.

Morris, D., Ward, A. W. M., and Handyside, A. J. (1968). Early discharge after hernia repair. *Lancet*, **1**, 681–4.

Piachaud, D. and Weddell, J. M. (1972). The economics of treating varicose veins. *Int. J. Epidemiol.*, **1** (3), 287–94.

Russell, E. M. (1974). *Patient costing study*. Scottish Health Services Studies No. 31. Scottish Home and Health Department.

Russell, I. T., Devlin, H. B., Fell, M., Glass, N. J., and Newell, D. J. (1977). Day case surgery for hernias and haemorrhoids: a clinical, social and economic evaluation. *Lancet*, **i**, 844–7.

Schneider, J. and Twiggs, L. B. (1972). The costs of carcinoma of the cervix. *Obstet. Gynaecol.*, **40** (6), 851–9.

Schweitzer, S. O. (1974). Cost effectiveness of early detection of disease. *Hlth Services Res.*, **9**, 22–32.

Shapiro, S. *et al.* (1973). Changes in 5 year breast cancer mortality in a breast cancer screening program. *Seventh National Cancer Conference Proceedings*.

Torrance, G. W., Sackett, D. L., and Thomas, W. H. (1973). Utility maximisation model for program evaluation: a demonstration application. In *Health status indexes* (ed. R. L. Berg). Hospital Research and Educational Trust, Chicago.

Venet, L., Strax, P., Venet, W., and Shapiro, S. (1971). Adequacies and inadequacies of breast examinations by physicians in mass screening. *Cancer*, **28** (6), 1546–51.

Wager, R. (1972). *Care of the elderly—an exercise in cost benefit analysis commissioned by Essex County Council*. I.M.T.A. (now Chartered Institute of Public Finance and Accountancy), London.

Williams, A. H. and Anderson, R. (1975). *Efficiency in the social services*. Basil Blackwell and Martin Robertson, London.

Williams, R. G. A., Johnston, M., Willis, L. A., and Bennet, A. E. (1976). Disability—a model and measurement technique. *Brit. J. prevent. soc. Med.*, **30**, 71–8.

Wright, K. G. (1974). Alternative measures of the output of social programmes: the elderly. In *Economic policies and social goals* (ed. A. J. Culyer). Martin Robertson, London.

—— (1978). Output measurement in practice. In *Economic aspects of health services* (ed. A. J. Culyer and K. G. Wright). Martin Robertson, London.

8
How useful is economic appraisal in health care?

The preceding chapters have illustrated the steps involved in undertaking economic appraisals in the field of health care. In the course of this exposition many practical difficulties have been identified and it is clear that economic appraisals are unlikely to give the decision-maker the answer to all his questions. In addition, it must be remembered that the appraisals themselves consume scarce resources, which, using the arguments set out in this book, could be used to provide care rather than to appraise it! Therefore, it is essential to pose the question, 'How useful is economic appraisal in health care?'

First, it is important to note that, although this book has been concerned primarily with the methodology to be employed in undertaking empirical cost-benefit studies, there can be consider-able benefit from using the same methodology merely as a *way of thinking* or as a *way of questioning current practice*. It is not costly (in relation to the potential benefits) to ask pertinent questions when resource allocation decisions are being made. Thus, one may ask:

Have all the resource consequences of this action been presented?
What are the likely benefits to patients?
Can these be measured?
What are the value judgements implied by the policy?
Whose values are they?

It may well be advantageous to insist on some further data collection if the answers to some of these questions are unclear in situations where it is important to be accurate (e.g. in the case of decisions where large amounts of resources are at stake) and where relevant data are believed to exist or could be readily assembled. (A more extensive list of the circumstances in which cost–benefit studies are likely to be beneficial was given in §4.4.)

Regardless of the scope for empirical study, there appear to be three aspects of economic appraisal that are potentially beneficial to clear thinking. First, it embodies a systematic approach to decision-making, as opposed to 'muddling through', and thus enables decision-makers to test the implications of each decision against all the objectives that they set themselves.

Second, economic appraisal recognizes the scarcity of resources and the principle that decisions should depend upon benefits foregone as well as benefits obtained. Given scarcity, a purely technical or medical frame of reference is no longer sufficient. Therefore, any form of appraisal proposed as an alternative to economic appraisal should have a similarly wide and rigorous perspective.

Third, economic appraisal offers a framework in which value judgements can be made explicit. There is no objective way of making policy decisions, merely more systematic ways of articulating the judgements involved.

Of course, the use of economic appraisal does have potential disadvantages which need to be guarded against. For example, there is the possibility that those elements in the appraisal which are difficult to measure are, in consequence, forgotten. Hence the need to keep the enumeration, measurement, and explicit valuation stages separate in the appraisal. In addition, there is the possibility that the decision-maker could be led to believe that the results of an economic appraisal give the total basis for a decision. Hence the need to consider criteria such as equity and the need (as in Chapter 6) to play down the mechanistic use of 'decision rules'. There is no simple, single basis for community-wide choices and the key to 'better' decisions lies in the interaction among the various forms of explicit analysis (like economic appraisal) and the decision-making process itself. The question is whether economic appraisal provides a useful way of organizing thought, not whether it could ever become a substitute for it.

Appendix 1

Economic appraisal in the context of clinical decision-making

In Chapter 1, it was stated that this book is primarily aimed at those individuals concerned with choice between alternatives in the context of *planning* health services. This would include not only those involved in health care planning in the institutional sense (e.g. community physicians, administrators, treasurers, and nurse administrators) but also those undertaking clinical trials of the 'pragmatic' attitude.[†] Many resource allocation decisions are made in the planning context.

However, at the other end of the spectrum there is the individual clinical practitioner (e.g. doctor, nurse, social worker) dealing with individual clients. The practitioner makes resource allocation decisions also. To what extent are the economic concepts set out in the book relevant to this resource allocation process?

What are the differences between decision-making in the planning and the clinical contexts?

There are two differences, both stemming from the fact that planning decisions are made for a group of people, whereas clinical decisions are typically made on behalf of one individual. The first difference is in the presentation of the *information* used in making the decision. In the planning context one is typically interested in aggregate information: which therapy is most effective on average; which therapy has the lowest cost on average? Moreover, it is obvious that the treatment which is the most effective or least costly for the group as a whole need not be the most effective or least costly for each individual concerned; for example, one might find that day-case surgery is less costly (on average) than traditional in-patient surgery for a particular condition. Therefore, given equal effectiveness of the two alternatives, one might argue on the whole for day-case surgery. Nevertheless, one might find that in some instances, the home circumstances of patients are such that they will require a great deal of support from community services. For these patients, day-case surgery may be the *more* costly alternative.

In the clinical context, the emphasis is on information particular to the individual patient or client. The object is to ascertain how that individual

---

† This terminology is after Schwartz and Lellouch (1967). Trials of the *pragmatic* attitude are those which aim at a choice between two alternative therapies for the given study population. This contrasts with clinical trials of an *explanatory* attitude, which seek merely to investigate the effects of a particular therapy.

will fare under the alternative regimens. The emphasis is often on a distribution of probability of effectiveness or cost rather than on the mean (or average). This attitude is implicit in the commonly expressed view that 'every patient is different'.

Closer inspection shows this difference between the planning and clinical perspectives to be reconcilable. It is true that in the planning context one does advise for the group, and, depending on the heterogeneity of the group, the best strategy for the group may not be the best strategy for each and every individual. However, there is scope within the planning context for a finer definition of the group in question. For instance, instead of advising two alternative treatments (say) for hernia sufferers as a whole, it would be possible to advise between the alternatives for different sub-groups, according to severity of condition, home circumstances, nature of employment, and any other factors likely to affect the success or cost of treatment. It is clear that, at the limit, the information sought in arriving at a decision would be similar in the planning and clinical contexts.

Nevertheless, there is another important difference between the two contexts that is not so easily reconcilable. This concerns the *value system* used in arriving at decisions. The notion underpinning this book is that the relevant group in arriving at health care planning decisions is the whole community. Although, at any one time, one might be comparing two alternative treatments for only a subset of the community (say the elderly), one would be implicitly considering the whole community if the costs and benefits of the alternatives were calculated along the lines set out in the book. This is because 'cost' has been taken to refer to the benefit forgone when units of a scarce resource are used. Thus the community as a whole *is* considered, since the 'cost' of the treatment under consideration is the value that members of the community place on the forgone benefit. It is suggested in this guide that the appropriate way to choose between alternatives on economic grounds in the planning context is to undertake a (*social*) cost–benefit analysis. That is, to calculate the costs and benefits falling on, or accruing to, all members of the community from each alternative course of action.

However, in the clinical context one could argue that the practitioner's sole concern is with his or her patient or client. It is still possible to undertake a cost–benefit analysis, but it will be a *private* cost-benefit analysis, on the client's behalf. For example, in weighing the pros and cons of treatment alternatives, the client's preferences for one therapy or another may be elicited (e.g. in terms of pain and restriction of activity or the relative financial losses, through loss of work time or travel expenses). Of course, the community at large may have an interest in some of these factors too—lost work time may imply lost production—but, generally speaking, the practitioner will not feel bound to consider that proportion of the cost or benefit of treatment which does not affect the client.

Nevertheless, it is worth noting that departures from the individual-based value system can be observed even in clinical practice. For instance, the practitioner may sometimes consider the costs and benefits falling on the client's family. This may be particularly true when the interests of the client and his (or her) family are in conflict. This may occur, for example, in the choice between domiciliary and institutional care for the elderly. Here the practitioner may arrive at a decision through (implicitly) undertaking a 'social cost–benefit analysis' for the 'community' consisting of the client *and* the family.

Another example of a departure from the individual-based value system is in the allocation of those scarce resources totally under the practitioner's control—for example, the allocation of the practitioner's own work time. Here the value of the time given to one individual has to be weighed against the time that will be given to others. In general terms the objective will be to maximize the value of the available time to the 'community' served. This is a rationing system akin to that suggested by the economic approach in the planning context.

Therefore it appears that economic concepts may have more applicability in the clinical context than would appear at first sight, particularly if the practitioner were to view himself as doing the 'best he can' for the 'community' of patients under his care. Suppose the practitioner were a surgeon, serving a 'community' consisting of patients on the waiting list plus those currently undergoing treatment. A shorter length of stay for some surgical procedures may result in some patients suffering a minor inconvenience (such as self-care for a short period after discharge), but it may also enable waiting time for surgery to be reduced. An investigation of the costs and benefits, to the individual practitioner's 'community', of an expansion of short-stay surgery would constitute a form of economic appraisal. It may, of course, be a little restricted in that the two alternative surgical strategies may have other resource implications outside the individual practitioner's immediate concern. For example, one might find that the short-stay alternative requires more diagnostic work, more nursing resources, or more medication. The individual practitioner may not look upon these as being scarce, since an increased consumption of them by some patients will not necessarily result in other patients in his 'community' going without treatment (or having to wait longer).

The approach outlined in this guide would include consideration of all the resources used in health treatments, since, taking the community as a whole, a benefit must be foregone somewhere whenever a scarce resource is used. The results of economic appraisals are likely therefore to be mainly the concern of planners, since it is they who must take a community-wide view. Remember that the group of 'planners' will include clinicians whenever they adopt that role—in becoming clinical members of management teams, in participating on medical committees, and in preparing requests for additional resources.

The extent to which an individual practitioner's own clinical practice is influenced by the results of full economic appraisals is likely to remain a matter for individual clinical freedom. However, there may be much that practitioners could do to improve the efficiency of their own practice for the benefit of their own 'community' of patients and in addition they may welcome more feedback on the wider resource consequences of clinical decisions. There are already signs that more practitioners are taking an interest in these issues and a number of Studies in the field of surgery are reported in Bunker, Barnes, and Mosteller (1977). In addition some of these studies are summarized in the companion volume, *Studies in economic appraisal in health care.*

REFERENCES

Bunker, J. P., Barnes, B. A., and Mosteller, F. eds. (1977). *Costs, risks and benefits of surgery.* Oxford University Press, New York.

Schwartz, D. and Lellouch, J. (1967). Explanatory and pragmatic attitudes in therapeutic trials *J. chron. Dis.*, **20**, 637–48.

Appendix 2

Distributive considerations in economic appraisal in health care

It is probably fair to say that, in undertaking economic appraisals in health care, economists have given relatively little attention to distributive considerations. To the economist, 'distribution' is shorthand for the 'distribution of income and wealth in the community'. This may not be completely the same as the health care professional's notion of distribution, and this point is taken up later.

A.2.1. How do distributive considerations affect economic appraisal?

There are two ways in which the distribution of income and wealth in the community impinge upon economic appraisal. First, the set of prices that we observe for goods and services derive from the market exchanges that are carried out given the existing distribution. Therefore, to the extent that the economist takes existing prices as a guide to costs and benefits he is tacitly 'accepting' the given distribution for the purposes of his study. However, it should be noted that economic appraisals in the health field tend to draw their values for costs and benefits from a wide variety of sources (see §4.3), and could be said to have departed somewhat from this position.

The second way in which distributive considerations impinge upon economic appraisal in the health field yields some suggestions for action. Health services are often seen either

(a) As an instrument for redistributing wealth in the community (that is, taxes are collected from the rich so that health services can be provided for all), or

(b) As a 'basic' commodity to which an individual's ability to pay should not restrict his access.

These two notions are probably related. The practical points emerging are that in the appraisal:

(a) One might want to discriminate in favour of low income groups in the provision of health care;

(b) One might not want willingness to pay to be a dominant feature in benefit measurements if willingness to pay is constrained by ability to pay.

A.2.2. How should one allow for distributive considerations in the appraisal?

The first step is to identify the incidence of costs and benefits of alternative programmes upon different income groups. If the distributive effects of the alternatives being appraised differ, this will then become apparent.

Following on from this, one could merely *display* the distributive effects, so that the decision-maker could take these into account along with the costs and benefits in total. Alternatively, one could derive a set of *distributive weights* to be incorporated in the appraisal. That is, £1 to a rich man would be weighted at less than £1 to a poor man. The question then arises of how to arrive at the weights. Economists have used two approaches. The first is to look for evidence of such relative weights elsewhere in society; for instance in the tax system. In direct taxation the higher one's income, the higher one's (marginal) tax rate. Therefore the marginal tax rates could be used to weight costs and benefits between different income groups: e.g. £1 to someone paying no tax would be weighted by unity, a benefit to someone paying tax at 30 per cent would be weighed by the factor 0.7. The second approach is to ask decision-makers to give the weights to be used in the appraisal. This has the advantage over the *display* approach, in that if forces the decision-maker to consider distributive consequences explicitly and systematically. However, in practice decision-makers are likely to find this difficult.

Mention of decision-makers raises the question of whether distribution is seen merely in income terms by health service decision-makers. Certainly one observes more discussion of distribution in terms of geographical area or in terms of client group. In many cases they may amount to the same thing—some client groups will be (on average) poorer than others, as will some geographical areas. Thinking of distribution in these terms has the attraction that it is congruent with the way services are provided, and the distributive issues can be shelved. For example, once it has been decided how much of total resources should be devoted (say) to the care of the elderly, one could examine alternative ways of caring for that group, setting aside the distributive question. This approach may be satisfactory up to a point, but it should be remembered that some elderly people are very rich and well able to provide for their own care. Also, it was 'discovered' in the recent debate over plans to redistribute health care resources in England that, although London was 'rich' in resources, some areas of London were 'deprived'.

FURTHER READING ON DISTRIBUTION

Walsh, H. G. and Williams, A. H. (1969). Current issues in cost–benefit analysis. *CAS Occasional Paper No. 11.* HMSO, London.

Williams, A. H. (1977). Income distribution and public expenditure decisions. In *Public expenditure* (ed. M. Posner). Cambridge University Press.

Appendix 3

The valuation of health states

This subject is worthy of a book on its own. Indeed there are already a number of texts dealing with the conceptual issues involved, the theoretical basis for the methodologies employed, and practical applications. Therefore I do not intend to go over the same ground in detail, but to outline the key features of approaches to the valuation of health states, so that these can be followed up in the additional reading indicated at the end of this appendix. In addition, two further points are discussed in order to build a bridge between the general issues of economic appraisal and medical evaluation discussed in this book, and the health status literature. These are (a) the valuation of health states as a logical extension of the assessment of medical effectiveness, and (b) the valuation of health states in the context of the cost–benefit approach.

A.3.1. The valuation of health states as an extension of the assessment of medical effectiveness

Suppose one were comparing the effectiveness of alternative treatments for a given acute condition. A number of indicators of the relative 'success' of the two treatments could be considered—for example, 'immediate' indicators, such as case fatality rate and complication rate, 'long-term' indicators, such as 5-year survival rate and recurrence rate. Whilst all these are relevant from the economist's point of view, since they all relate to the benefits or to the costs of care, a number of problems in interpretation can arise. First, it may be that one treatment may not be superior on all counts—for example, it may have a higher case fatality rate but better long-term characteristics for survivors.

Second, the 'outputs' to which indicators relate may not be homogeneous—one complication may be more serious than another; a year of life gained by one treatment mode may be of lower quality than that gained by another.

Clearly the assessment of the 'success' of alternative therapies is often ambiguous and will require more than just the recording of information such as the 'number of complications'. Often the discussion can be broadened by a description of the *types* of complications experienced or the *type* of life that the patient can lead *post*-treatment: e.g. whether or not the patient can return to his original employment or to an alternative employment; whether or not he can take regular holidays; whether or not he can hold a driving licence. This more detailed discussion may aid the assessment of the success of the treatment alternatives.

If this discussion were to be taken further it would emerge that three sets of questions need to be answered in making an assessment of the relative success of therapies or programmes. These are:

1. *What constitutes health or ill-health?* Health can be defined in several different ways. The World Health Organization (1948) defines health as 'a state of complete physical, mental and social well-being, and not merely the absence of disease or infirmity'. Twaddle (1974) suggests that from a biological standpoint 'perfect health' might be seen as 'a state in which every cell of the body is functioning at optimum capacity and in perfect harmony with each other cell'. This contrasts with a definition from a social standpoint where 'perfect health may be a state in which an individual's capacities for taste and role performance are optimised'. In the literature on the valuation of health states, there has been an emphasis upon the specification of particular 'dimensions' of health along which changes can be measured: e.g. two dimensions frequently specified are pain and degree of restriction of activity (see Mooney 1979; Williams 1974). See also the examples given in the case studies on chronic renal failure and care of the elderly. It is easy to see how the specification of 'complications' could be encompassed within this latter approach, since one of the features of a 'complication' is that it is likely to affect some aspect of the patient's physical, mental, or social functioning either in the present or in the future.

2. *How are the various components of health or ill-health valued relative to one another?* Inevitably, the assessment of treatment alternatives involves the consideration of the relative importance of, say, avoiding one type of complication as against another, or the consideration of, say, the pros and cons of a higher risk treatment with better long-term prospects, versus one with the opposite characteristics.

3. *At what time do the various events occur and for how long do they last?*

The research work in the field of health status indexes has tackled these very issues. Its main contribution has been to systematize our thinking in this very difficult area. The key features of existing approaches are outlined below.

A.3.2. Key features in approaches to the valuation of health states

It is best to view the valuation of health states as a step-wise process, each step employing technical judgements and/or value judgements. The key stages in all approaches are:

(a) The specification of the main dimensions in which health state is to be measured.

(b) The scaling, and hence measurement, of positions (or states) along the specified dimensions.

(c) The relative valuation of *combinations* of characteristics in the specified dimensions.

(d) The absolute valuation of the combinations.

If movements in the health status index are to be compared with the costs of the programmes required to produce those movements, there is a further stage, involving the specification of the 'worth' of those movements in money terms (see §A.3.3). However, this section concentrates on stages (a) to (d).

The specification of the dimensions along which health state is to be measured amounts to a specification of the objectives of the treatments or health policies in question. It should be noted that this is a value judgement which, by and large, is made by health professionals. One result of the research into health status measurement is that this value judgement is more widely recognized and the appropriate source of the values more widely discussed.

The scaling and measurement of movements along the specified dimensions is usually a complicated process involving both technical and value judgements. For example, suppose that the *maintenance of independence* is one of the dimensions along which improvements in the health of, say, the elderly is to be measured. This could be expressed in terms of the elderly person's mobility and ability to perform a number of key tasks, such as washing, dressing, feeding, and so on. The list could be endless and a way has to be found of reducing the number of components. Several statistical methods (such as correlation and factor analysis) and lexicographic scaling techniques (such as Guttman Scaling) have been applied. (See Culyer 1978; Wright 1978.) The main pitfall seems to be associated with an unthinking movement into simple scoring techniques, which may lead to the naïve interpretation that by adding the scores one is able to say that one combination of disabilities is 'so many times worse' than another. The main error implicit in this approach is that one needs to allow for the possibility that a *combination* of disabilities is worse than the sum of each considered separately. For this reason and for others, a number of researchers have been content with the production of an *ordinal* scaling of states along each dimension, leaving matters of cardinality to the later stages in the development of the health status index.

If it is possible to obtain ordinal scales giving the states of health or ill-health along each dimension, the next stage is to obtain relative and absolute valuations of *combinations* of states, comprising of one state from each of the dimensions. The majority of the methods employed to date have been similar in that they present the judge with descriptions of the combinations of states and ask him to choose between them in a way that allows quantification of his choices. Culyer (1978) identifies five main methods in the existing health status literature. Some methods ask the judge directly to score particular health states relative to a given standard. Another method obtains a linear ranking of states by presenting the judge with a choice between a certainty of being in one health state and a 'gamble' of being worse off or better off. In a third method the judge is asked what length of time x in the healthy state would be equivalent to a longer time t in a dysfunctional state, assuming death would immediately follow in each case. Each of the methods has its own rationale and the reader is advised to consult the detailed descriptions given in Culyer (1978) and in the original research publications. Some practical examples of this type of work were given in Chapter 7. Most of the valuation methods simultaneously combine the trading off of component dimensions of health and the assignment of over-all scores to the health state combinations.

A.3.3. The valuation of health states in the context of the cost–benefit approach

The economic researcher could find himself confronting the issues outlined above irrespective of whether his original intention was to undertake a cost benefit analysis or to undertake a cost effectiveness analysis.

In a full cost–benefit analysis an attempt is made to express all the relevant costs and benefits in commensurate units—this is normally taken to mean money terms. However, this may prove to be very difficult and it may be decided to express only changes in resource use and changes in productive output in money terms. A first step towards comparing all the costs and benefits of alternative programmes would than be to measure the changes in health state obtained in each and to set these against the net costs of the programmes. One way of taking the analysis further would than be to value the changes in health state gained, not in money terms, but in index form. In fact, using the reasoning employed in Chapter 4 (§4.4) one could argue that the fact that choices *are* made implies that this type of valuation is always made subconsciously. In an ideal world all the health improvements gained from all treatments would be expressed in terms of multiples of a common 'health unit' and the health budget would then be allocated so as to maximize the number of health units gained in each year.†

Although the cost–*benefit* analyst may find himself considering the valuation of health states, it is much more likely that the route to these issues will be via cost *effectiveness* analysis. It will be remembered from Chapter 3 (§3.1) that the simple cost effectiveness approach can only be applied when the two alternatives produce an equivalent medical outcome or when there is one clear objective of medical intervention and the 'success' of that intervention can be measured unambiguously. In situations where these conditions do not hold, the valuation of health states provides one way combining multidimensional 'success' data into a single index of achievements, the changes in which can be compared subsequently with the relative costs of programmes. In this case, obtaining valuations of health states is equivalent to assigning 'weights' to the achievements of particular treatment objectives.

A.3.4. Summary

(a) The field of activity reviewed in this appendix is still largely experimental in its nature.

(b) The methodologies employed provide no 'magical answer' to the

---

† Adjusted for any distributional considerations, of course. See Appendix 2.

difficult choices involved in allocating health care resources. Rather they provide a method of identifying the crucial elements in making the choices, so that these can be considered in turn.

(c) These choices will remain irrespective of whether more effort is put into the derivation of health status indexes. The most immediate outcome of more work may not be that the choices appear 'easier' but that those concerned are forced to give more explicit consideration to the various technical and value questions raised.

REFERENCES

Culyer, A. J. (1978). Need, values and health status measurement. In *Economic aspects of health services* (ed. A. J. Culyer and K. G. Wright). Martin Robertson, London.

Mooney, G. H. (1979). Values in health care. In *Economics and health planning* (ed. K. Lee). Croom Helm, London.

Twaddle, A. C. (1974). The concept of health status. *Social Sci. Med.*, **8**, 29–38.

World Health Organisation (1948). Official Records No. 2, June.

Williams, A. H. (1974). Measuring the effectiveness of health care systems. *Brit. J. prevent. soc. Med.*, **28** (3), 196–202.

Wright, K. G. (1978). Output measurement in practice. In *Economic aspects of health services* (ed. A. J. Culyer and K. G. Wright). Martin Robertson, London.

FURTHER READING

Introduction to the concepts

Culyer, A. J. (1976). *Need and the National Health Service*, Chapter 4. Martin Robertson, London.

More detailed discussion of theory and practice

Berg, R. L. (Ed.) (1973). *Health status indexes.* Hospital Research and Educational Trust, Chicago.

Culyer, A. J. (1978). *Measuring health: lessons for Ontario.* University of Toronto Press for Ontario Economic Council, Toronto.

Rosser, R. M. and Watts, V. C. (1974). The development of a classification of the symptoms of illness and its use to measure the output of a hospital. In *Impairment, disability and handicap* (ed. D. Lees and S. Shaw). Heinemann for SSRC, London.

Appendix 4

Discounting

A.4.1. The social rate of discount

What is the appropriate rate of discount to use in the appraisal of public sector investments—such as the provision of health care? Economists have debated this question at length. Market interest rates may give some indication of the premium that individuals require in order to postpone the satisfaction of their current wants. However, it is often argued that these are inappropriate for a number of reasons. In particular:

1. They may incorporate an element of risk which is not present in public sector investment.
2. The community may take a different view of the future when behaving *collectively* from that which it takes when behaving as individuals. (Many of us may have a vague feeling that this generation should provide for future generations, although as individuals we may behave as through the world is going to end tomorrow!)

Therefore, it is often argued that the *social rate of time preference* will be lower than observed market rates. One could view it as reflecting the current generation's preferences regarding the distribution of resources between itself and future generations. Thus, it is often suggested that a lower discount rate should be employed in the discounting procedure, but there is disagreement as to how much lower it should be.

One way out of this dilemma is suggested by an alternative approach to the derivation of a public sector discount rate. This starts from the premise that at any moment in time there will be a limit to the funds available for investment. Under these circumstances, one extra public sector investment means that investment opportunities elsewhere in the economy (say, in the private sector) will have to be forgone. Using this *opportunity cost* argument, it is suggested that the appropriate public sector discount rate is one which would ensure that public sector investment does not displace any private sector investment offering the community a higher net social benefit. Thus, it is argued that the public sector should be applying a 'test' discount rate on its investment appraisals, to ensure equivalence at the margin with practice in the private sector. Application of a single test discount rate would also ensure equivalence, at the margin, within different segments of the public sector.

The choice of social rate of discount can be seen to be a complex matter. Is private sector investment displaced at the margin? Are the funds for public sector investment drawn from private households (e.g. by taxation) and thereby displacing individuals' consumption? These factors may be difficult to identify. However, in practice the choice of discount rate is simplified for the individual analyst, since a rate is often promulgated from the centre. In the UK the Treasury advised a rate of 10 per cent between 1969 and 1978, reduced in that year to 7 per cent.

A.4.2. A worked example

The first step in discounting is to identify the time at which costs and benefits occur. In the example below, it is assumed that costs and benefits can be depicted as single amounts occurring at one-yearly intervals. Suppose that it is mid-1978† now, and the first costs and benefits occur. The next costs and benefits (in mid-1979) are one year away, and so on. In principle there is nothing to stop one considering costs and benefits occurring, say, on a monthly basis, although the calculation will be slightly more complicated. No costs or benefits occur after 1982 in this example.

	1978	1979	1980	1981	1982	
Alternative A						
Costs (£)	300	50	50	50	50	
Benefits (£)	100	150	200	200	200	
(Benefits − costs)	− 200	100	150	150	150	Σ(Benefits − costs) = £350

	1978	1979	1980	1981	1982	
Alternative B						
Costs (£)	300	100	100	0	0	
Benefits (£)	250	300	200	50	50	
(Benefits − costs)	− 50	200	100	50	50	Σ(Benefits − costs) = £350

It can be seen that both the alternatives produce an undiscounted excess of benefits over costs of £350. In order to discount, each year's total must be multiplied by the factor

$$\frac{1}{(1 + r)^n},$$

where $r =$ the rate of discount (say 10 per cent) and $n =$ the number of years into the future.

† The mid-point of the year is taken for convenience only. Equally, the beginning of each year could have been taken.

Therefore we have for alternative A:

Present value of (benefits − costs) (i.e. net present value (NPV) in £) =

$$-200\frac{1}{(1+0.1)^0} + 100\frac{1}{(1+0.1)^1} + 150\frac{1}{(1+0.1)^2}$$

$$+150\frac{1}{(1+0.1)^3} + 150\frac{1}{(1+0.1)^4}$$

NPV(£) = −200 + 100(0.91) + 150(0.84) + 150(0.77) + 150(0.70)
    = −200 + 91 + 126 + 115.5 + 105
NPV(£) = 237.5.

Similarly for alternative B:

Net present value (£) = −50 + 200(0.91) + 100(0.84) + 50(0.77)
        + 50(0.70)
NPV(£) = −50 + 182 + 84 + 38.5 + 35
NPV(£) = 289.5.

Therefore it can be seen that, far from being indifferent between the two alternatives, one would prefer alternative B in present value terms. We can see why if we return to the raw data. Under alternative B the majority of the net benefits accrue towards the beginning of the project period, whilst with alternative A the majority of the net benefits accrue towards the end of the project period. A positive discount rate implies a preference for benefits now, rather than benefits in the future.

Appendix 5

Some practical hints†

A.5.1. Finding an economist

If, after reading this guide, you decide that you would like the specialist help of an economist, it is important to involve him or her at the early stages of research design—in the same way that it is important to involve the statistician at the design stage of a clinical trial. In a number of countries, economists (and others) with an interest in health economics have formed associations, in order to enable members with like interests to maintain contact with each other. In the United Kingdom the association is called the *Health Economists' Study Group* and is supported financially by the Social Science Research Council. The organizer of the Group will be able to provide you with a list of the names and addresses of members, along with details of their current activities in research and teaching. In this way it will be possible to locate health economists near to your own place of work and/or economists working on problems similar to the one that you propose to tackle. Enquiries should be forwarded to:

The Organizer,
SSRC Health Economists' Study Group,
Institute of Social and Economic Research,
University of York,
Heslington,
York YO1 5DD.

In the event that an enquiry to the Health Economists' Study Group proves unfruitful, an alternative would be to contact the DHSS or SSRC. In their role as grant awarding bodies for health economics or related research, these organizations have acquired knowledge of the research workers active in the field.

Enquiries should be addressed to:

(a) *DHSS*
Economic Adviser's Office (Health),
Department of Health and Social Security,
Friars House,
157 Blackfriars Road,
LONDON SE1.

† These apply primarily to those living and working in the UK but it is hoped that others will find them useful.

(b) *SSRC*
The Secretary,
Executive Panel on Health and Health Policy,
Social Science Research Council,
1 Temple Avenue,
LONDON EC4Y 0BD.

A.5.2. Locating the relevant data

A.5.2.1. Changes in health service resources
The most important data here are those contained in the *Health Service Cost Returns*.

Following the reorganization of the NHS, new costing arrangements were set out for hospital services, community health services, the ambulance service, family practitioner service, and the blood transfusion service. Cost returns are made every year and can be obtained from the finance department of the relevant tier of the service e.g. hospital returns are held at the District, ambulance returns at the Region.

The returns represent an important source of cost data and should always be located. The main difficulties in using them to obtain the costs of alternative treatments are as follows:

1. *They are incomplete*—some parts of the Service do not produce all the information requested on the forms.
2. *They are highly aggregated*—e.g. hospital costs are generally broken down by in-patients, out-patients, and Accident and Emergency, and by hospital department. They are not usually broken down by treatment specialty or by type of treatment.
3. *They are average costs* (see comments in Chapters 4 and 7 on the distinction between average and marginal costs).
4. *They do not include capital costs.* If the changes in resource use brought about by the alternatives being assessed include changes in the use of buildings or equipment, additional costs will need to be included.

These 4 points indicate that routine cost returns are normally the starting point for the assessment of the costs of alternative treatments, rather than the finishing point.

A.5.2.2. Changes in other community resources
Important data sources for cost or benefit estimation here are:

1. Cost returns of any of the public and private bodies involved, e.g. local authorities, voluntary organizations. These are likely to suffer from many of the problems outlined in §A.5.2.1.
2. Values of individuals' time imputed in other empirical economic studies. (Ask your economist about this.)
3. Expenditure by families on health care, including the provision of

'hotel' services such as accommodation, food, heating, and lighting. Much of this information is unlikely to be available on a routine basis, but the *Family expenditure survey* and *Social trends*† are good general sources.

A.5.2.3. Changes in productive output

Earnings of patients and their relatives, are the most important data here. For a particular group of patients this is unlikely to be available on a routine basis, but the *Department of Employment Gazette*‡ gives aggregate information on wage rates, hours, and earnings for various occupations.

A.5.2.4. Changes in health state

The most important data sources here are:

1. *The results of medical evaluations;*
2. *Implied valuations of health outputs.* For example, see the table of implied valuations of human life in Mooney (1977, pp. 159–61), court awards, and the results of empirical research, such as that reported in Berg (1973).
3. Clearing House on Health Status Indicators, US Department of Health, Education, and Welfare, Public Health Service, 5600 Fishers Lane, Rockville, Maryland 20857, USA.

REFERENCES

Berg, R. L. (Ed.) (1973). *Health status indexes.* Hospital Research and Education Trust, Chicago.
Mooney, G. H. (1977). *The valuation of human life.* Macmillan, London.

† *Family Expenditure Survey*, Department of Employment, published annually by HMSO. *Social Trends*, Central Statistical Office, also published annually by HMSO.
‡ *Department of Employment Gazette* published monthly by HMSO.

Appendix 6

The use of earnings data in economic appraisals in health care

Patients' earnings may often be taken into account by the clinician in arriving at treatment decisions. In deciding upon the appropriate regimen for a given patient, he might select the regimen (all else being equal) that minimizes the patient's earnings loss. Furthermore, the fact that some patients may be losing income while waiting for treatment may be one factor in deciding upon treatment priorities. Here the emphasis is on the personal loss to the patient, resulting either from a prolonged wait for treatment or from work time lost as a result of treatment. The relevant cash sum would be the patient's wage net of tax, less any sickness benefit payments. However, the use of earnings data by economists has had a different focus and it is worthwhile discussing this to remove any ambiguity.

In the early cost–benefit studies, the use of earnings data reflected a very narrow view of the economic benefits of health programmes. That is, the value of an individual to the community was represented by the present value of the goods or services that he could produce during his working life. If a health programme increased this, through reducing morbidity or mortality, the benefits were represented by the discounted sum of the extra earnings gained. This is sometimes referred to as the *human capital approach* to the calculation of the benefits of health service investments. A major assumption of the approach is that the value of the goods and services produced is reflected in the individual's wages.

A variant of this approach argues that where a fatality is averted by the health service investment, the discounted earnings should be taken *net* of the individual's consumption since, upon his death, the community loses not only his production but also his consumption. Therefore, for a person who consumes exactly what he produces the net loss to the community from his death is zero. However, a strong argument against this approach is that *ex ante*, when the decision to invest is being taken, the person who would otherwise die is alive and a member of the community. Therefore, the loss of his consumption is a relevant factor in the consideration of the potential benefits from the investment (see Dowie (1970) for a more rigorous treatment of this).

This approach to the estimation of benefits (and, conversely, the estimation of the cost to the community of illness) is no longer upheld by economists, as it is clear that there are much wider economic benefits resulting from health programmes. (These were discussed more fully in

§4.1.) Nevertheless, earnings data can give a guide to the production losses and gains associated with health programmes, and it is in this sense that they are included in the approach recommended here.† When using earnings data for this purpose it is important to bear in mind the following points.

1. The use of earnings data represents a market-based approach to valuation and is therefore subject to all the reservations set out in §4.3.1.
2. Earnings data usually relate to average changes rather than marginal changes. Therefore, short absences from work may not result in production losses of the value indicated by wages.
3. It may be the job, or the position, that has the productive capacity rather than the individual. Therefore, if the individual is replaced by someone else, the final effect of his removal from the work-force may be just that one more person is removed from the ranks of the unemployed. Thus the final loss to the community may be much less than the earnings attracted by the position occupied by the individual originally removed. It may be much closer to zero—the opportunity cost of using unemployed labour.
4. Care should be taken to avoid double counting where earnings are used in conjunction with patients' valuations of the treatment received. This is because in making his assessment of the value to him of treatment, the individual may allow for the fact that it will enable him to retain consumption capacity which he otherwise would have lost.

REFERENCES

Dowie, J. A. (1970). Valuing the benefit of health improvement. *Australian Economic Papers*, June, 21–41.

† Here, the relevant earnings figures are gross earnings, plus employment taxes. Neither sickness benefits nor taxation enter the calculation.

Index